A TEXTBOOK OF INDUSTRIAL PHARMACY II

AS PER THE LATEST SYLLABUS PRESCRIBED BY PCI
FOR BACHELOR OF PHARMACY (B.PHARM) COURSE

DR. SHIKHA BAGHEL CHAUHAN

Made with ♥ on the Notion Press Platform
www.notionpress.com

Contents

Preface

INDUSTRIAL PHARMACY II Book for B. Pharm VII Semester 4th year (As per PCI Regulations).

The Industrial Pharmacy II Book [BP 702 T] is designed for B. Pharm VII Sem (B.Pharm 4th year) students and is strictly as per the Pharmacy Council of India (PCI) regulations.

Industrial Pharmacy II Book aims to impart fundamental knowledge on pharmaceutical product development and its journey from laboratory development to commercial scale production. Upon completion of the course, students shall be able to :

1. Know the process of pilot plant and scale up of pharmaceutical dosage forms
2. Understand the process of technology transfer from lab scale to commercial batch
3. Know different Laws and Acts that regulate pharmaceutical industry
4. Understand the approval process and regulatory requirements for drug products

Industrial Pharmacy II relates different aspects of product formulation development covering the Pilot plant scale up techniques, Technology development and transfer. Its also provides insights of regulatory affairs and regulatory requirments for drug approval. The book covers and discusses Quality managment systems and Indian regulatoty requirements.

It describes each and every topic in simplified way and at the same time provides the information and knowledge in depth. This book will be highly useful by B. Pharmacy VII Semester students.

The present book is an attempt to provide fundamental knowledge related to different aspects of Industrial Pharmacy II to the students. The subject matter has been presented in simple language supplemented with appropriate tables and figures, wherever required. The author would be grateful to receive suggestions for further improvement of the book.

Dr. Shikha Baghel Chauhan

Acknowledgements

It is our immense pleasure to publish and present this book of Industrial Pharmacy II to the pharmaceutical sciences students, teachers, and research scholars.

Any successful outcome is not an individual effort, but it is a joint venture of many people who put in their mind and soul for the completion of the work.

I would like to acknowledge the extraordinary debt I owe to my dear students Mansi sharma, Banaja swain, Vinita, Ishaan Aggarwal, Shallu singh and Suhani Rana. I would never have been able, to complete this book without their support and motivation.

I am pleased to express my deep sense of gratitude towards my parents for their constant encouragement and motivation to transform my teachings in the form of a user-friendly book for the students.

I am highly thankful to our Head of Institution, Dr. Sandeep Arora sir, for always providing support, motivation, and constant encouragement.

I hope this book will help the students in understanding the core concepts of subject and develop deep understanding of subject.

The readers of this book are requested to present their reviews and suggestions which will be highly appreciated and accepted by the authors. Constructive suggestions, comments and criticism on the subject matter of the book will be gratefully acknowledged, as they will certainly help to improve future editions of the book.

Syllabus

BP 702 T. INDUSTRIAL PHARMACY II (Theory)

UNIT-I

Pilot plant scale up techniques: General considerations - including significance of personnel requirements, space requirements, raw materials, Pilot plant scale up considerations for solids, liquid orals, semi solids and relevant documentation, SUPAC guidelines, Introduction to platform technology

UNIT-II

Technology development and transfer: WHO guidelines for Technology Transfer(TT): Terminology, Technology transfer protocol, Quality risk management, Transfer from R & D to production (Process, packaging and cleaning), Granularity of TT Process (API, excipients, finished products, packaging materials) Documentation, Premises and equipments, qualification and validation, quality control, analytical method transfer, Approved regulatory bodies and agencies, Commercialization - practical aspects and problems (case studies), TT agencies in India - APCTD, NRDC, TIFAC, BCIL, TBSE / SIDBI; TT related documentation - confidentiality agreement, licensing, MoUs, legal issues

UNIT-III

Regulatory affairs: Introduction, Historical overview of Regulatory Affairs, Regulatory authorities, Role of Regulatory affairs department, Responsibility of Regulatory Affairs Professionals

Regulatory requirements for drug approval: Drug Development Teams, Non-Clinical Drug Development, Pharmacology, Drug Metabolism and Toxicology, General considerations of Investigational New Drug (IND) Application, Investigator's Brochure (IB) and New Drug Application (NDA), Clinical research / BE studies, Clinical Research Protocols, Biostatistics in Pharmaceutical Product Development, Data Presentation for FDA Submissions, Management of Clinical Studies.

UNIT-IV

Quality management systems: Quality management & Certifications: Concept of Quality, Total Quality Management, Quality by Design (QbD), Six Sigma concept, Out of Specifications (OOS), Change control, Introduction to ISO 9000 series of quality systems standards, ISO 14000, NABL, GLP

UNIT-V

Indian Regulatory Requirements: Central Drug Standard Control Organization (CDSCO) and State Licensing Authority: Organization, Responsibilities, Certificate of Pharmaceutical Product (COPP), Regulatory requirements and approval procedures for New Drugs.

Author's Affiliations

Ms Mansi sharma (Chapter 1), B.Pharm, Amity Institute of Pharmacy, Amity University, Noida, Uttar Pradesh, India 201303

Ms Banaja swain (Chapter 2), M.Pharm, Amity Institute of Pharmacy, Amity University, Noida, Uttar Pradesh, India 201303

Ms Vinita (Chapter 2), M.Pharm, Amity Institute of Pharmacy, Amity University, Noida, Uttar Pradesh, India 201303

Ms Suhani Rana (Chapter 3), B.Pharm, Amity Institute of Pharmacy, Amity University, Noida, Uttar Pradesh, India 201303

Mr Ishaan Aggarwal (Chapter 4), B.Pharm, Amity Institute of Pharmacy, Amity University, Noida, Uttar Pradesh, India 201303

Ms Shallu Singh (Chapter 5), M.Pharm, Amity Institute of Pharmacy, Amity University, Noida, Uttar Pradesh, India 201303

CHAPTER I

UNIT 1 Pilot Plant Scale Up Techniques

At the end of the chapter, student will understand and gain knowledge about :

Pilot plant scale up techniques

General considerations - including significance of personnel requirements, space requirements, raw materials, Pilot plant scale up considerations for solids, liquid orals, semi solids and relevant documentation, SUPAC guidelines, Introduction to platform technology

ABSTRACT

Abstract: In the pharmaceutical industry, a lab-scale formula is scaled up to a large scale by developing a reliable and practical manufacturing procedure. This process is known as pilot plant scale-up. Solid dosage form pilot plant scale-up procedures will offer manufacturing guidelines for large-scale processes and will be essential for large-scale production. A critical role will be played by general scale-up requirements like reporting responsibilities, personnel needs, workspace requirements, formula reviews, raw material processing equipment, production rates, and GMP considerations, as well as parameters like blending, granulation, drying, and compression. Compared to large-scale production facilities, pilot plants are typically smaller. The creation of many cGMP batches in the pilot-plants, which are also learning facilities, gives their staff the chance to follow and validate the procedure.

INTRODUCTION

The Pilot Plant is a Manufacturing and Hybrid Development Unit that incorporates the development, developmental activities in infancy, manufacturing of clinical supplies technology assessment, expansion and move to production locations.

A pilot-plant is in fact a pre-commercial producing system that produces in small quantities using novel production techniques and/or new technologies, typically with the intention of better understanding the latter. The gained knowledge is then applied to the design of industrial manufacturing systems and consumer products, as well as to the choice of future research directions and the justification of financial choices. Pilot plants are also often more adaptable because they are designed for learning, which may come at the sacrifice of the economy. Other pilot plants take significant engineering work, cost millions of dollars, and are made from process equipment, instrumentation, and pipes. Some pilot plants are constructed in laboratories using standard lab equipment. Additionally, they can be utilized to train workers for a real plant. Compared to demonstration plants, pilot plants are typically smaller.

Scaleup *is a method for applying the same process to various output quantities by*

increasing the batch size. Therefore, the process of developing and formulating process knowledge so that it may be used to effectively direct the selection of materials, operating parameters, processing parameters, and process control techniques, regardless of scale, is known as scale-up.

The current good manufacturing practices (cGMP) environment, highly competent employees, equipment support, and the ability to thoroughly and closely examine the formula are all required for the pilot plant investigations.

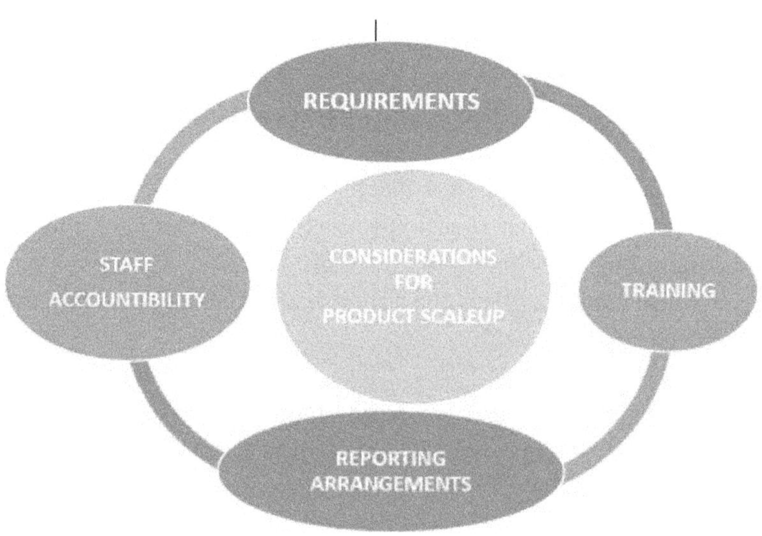

FIG.1: CONSIDERATIONS FOR SCALE-UP TECHNIQUE

Preparation for FDA pre-approval inspection.

-Key technical elements:

Major technological aspects that are in the early stages of development are included in the scaling up of the pilot plant.

Critical component control, critical component identification. Formulation variable identification, formula variable control, combining manufacturing regions, and equipment with those of the test plant, critical process parameter identification, identifying the equipment in the pilot plant's operational ranges, and gathering of process and product data.

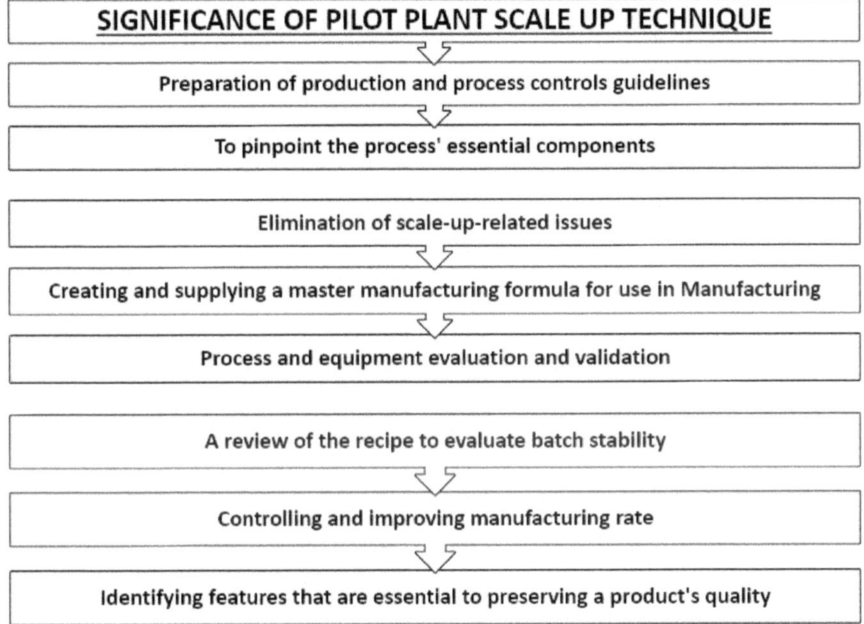

FIG.2: SIGNIFICANCE OF PILOT PLANT SCALE-UP TECHNIQUE

FACTORS AFFECTING PILOT PLANT SCALE-UP TECHNIQUE

1. Administration and information flow

I. Both scientists and technicians should have access to adequate office and desk space.
II. The area ought to be close to the workspace.
III. Computers.
IV. Physical testing area: This space ought to include a permanent bench top for equipment that is frequently utilized for physical testing.

2. Space Requirements

A pilot plant needs four different types of space

I. Processing information and administration tasks
To enable accurate documentation of the scientists' actions and observations, there should be enough office and desk space for both the scientists and technicians. It should be close to the workspace yet far enough away to prevent excessive distractions while people are working.

I. Area for Physical Testing: There should be an appropriate area in which samples could be actively checked and evaluated for in quality control assessment (which helps in the early discovery of production problems).. Permanent bench space for frequently used physical testing tools like balances, pH meters, viscometers, etc. should be provided in this area.

III. **Standard floor space for pilot plant equipment**

It has to do with where all the equipment used during the scale-up procedures at the pilot plant are kept. The machinery must be available in a variety of sizes that are familiar to the representation of all manufacturing capabilities. With this design, it is possible to ensure the accuracy of the scale-up data that is gathered while also using expensive materials to assess the effects of scale-up on research formulations and processes, intermediate size and large or full-scale manufacturing equipment are crucial. When at all practicable, equipment should be made portable because pilot plant equipment is irregular or intermittent and depends on project assignments. The best way to use this space is to divide it into sections for the various dose form.

3. Standard floor space for pilot plant equipment

I. The equipment required to manufacture all sorts of dosage forms is placed in a discrete pilot plant
II. Location or assess how well research formulations and methods scale up, full scale, and intermediate production equipment are required.
III. Wherever possible, equipment should be made portable. So that, it may be put away in the tiny storage area after usage.
IV. It should be possible to clean the equipment in a designated area.

4. Formula review

I. It's crucial to carefully examine the vitality content of the formulation process.
II. It is vital to comprehend the function of each ingredient and how it contributes to the finished product produced in small-scale laboratory machinery.
III. The impact of scaling up employing machinery that might subject the product to stresses of various kinds and intensities can then be foreseen or identified more easily.

5. Raw Materials

The active and excipient raw materials used in the formulation of pharmaceutical products must be approved and validated, which is one of the duties of the pilot plant because we wouldn't take it casually. This is due to the fact that a pilot scale-up alone cannot guarantee a seamless transformation.

The need for big volume shipments of materials used on a full manufacturing scale may not be met by the raw materials utilized during small-scale formulation studies. Additionally, as a product is scaled up, the active chemicals used on a laboratory scale must be able to fulfill the increasing demands of the product.

As the batch size grows, there may be variations in the density, static charges, rate of solubility, morphology, or flow properties of the active/inert ingredients, which could lead to varied handling properties. Alternative raw material providers are necessary because a lone supplier occasionally leaves the business unprotected in terms of price and supply quality. This calls for the production of numerous batches of products using these alternative components, with their formulation and final product stability performance being compared to the regular product.

6. Resources

I. The simplest, most cost-effective machinery that can produce goods that meet the requested criteria is used.
II. The equipment's size should be such that the experimental trials conducted apply to batches of the size as those used for production.
III. If the equipment is too huge, valuable active ingredients will be wasted, but if it is too small, the method established will not scale up.

IV. Cleaning ease.

7. Production Rates

When determining the production rates, both current and upcoming market trends and requirements are taken into account.

8. Parameters used in Process Evaluation

I. Order of component mixing, mixing time and speed,
II. The rate at which granulating agents, solvents, medicinal solutions, etc.
III. Rates for heating and cooling
IV. Size of filters (liquids)
V. Display size (solids)
VI. Drying temperature and duration

Limitations of scale-up technique

Challenges with scale-up

I. To address these issues, scale-up projects for pilot plants need to conduct numerous in-depth engineering studies.
II. Front-End In modeling software, engineering, and scale-up design should both be done during the design phase.
III. The constraints of your technology can be determined by modeling utilizing semi-empirical approaches.
IV. It should be demonstrated that the chemical method can be scaled up to achieve the desired result for a fair price until a finalized agreement is reached.

LIMITATIONS

SCALING UP NON LINEARLY	• Non-linear scaling is the primary barrier to scaling up a pilot plant and it also contributes to the other seven barriers. Non—-linear level, in its simplest form, means that you cannot simply proportionally increase the number of chemicals and equipment required to transfer a chemical method from a lab to a pilot plant..
REACTION STRATEGIES	• The particles in a process should mix well in order for equilibrium to b e reached as quickly as possible. • Poor reaction kinetics can result from inefficient mixing and collision, which can be caused by a variety of physical and chemical factors.
CHEMICAL STABILITY	• The reaction takes longer to reach chemical equilibrium when additional chemicals are added. For a reaction to be productive, chemical equilibrium must initially be reached.
MATERIAL ATTRIBUTES	• The chemical and physical properties of the substances in touch with t he reaction may have an impact on it, causing it to degrade over time, or unnecessarily raise the system's cost. So it's important to pick the co rrect material.
FLUID DYNAMICS	• Maintaining flow at the right Reynolds number is essential for efficient mixing and thermal transmission, but this number varies nonlinearly as systems get bigger. Laminar to turbulent flow transitions can be unpre dictable due to the non-linear nature of fluid dynamics.
THERMO-DYNAMICS	• To successfully scale up a chemical process, a thorough thermodynami c study is needed since chemical processes are sensitive to solar heat a nd heat loss

FIG.3: LIMITATIONS OF SCALE-UP TECHNIQUE

DESIGN FOR TABLETS PILOT-PLANT

The major responsibility of a pilot -plant staff would be to ensure that the recently developed tablets made by the product design team will demonstrate to be productively, reasonably priced, and continuously repeatable..The pharmaceuticals pilot plant in tablet development should be built with the features required for easy maintenance and hygiene. It should ideally be situated mostly on the ground floor to speed up supply delivery and shipping. In the lab, substances are simply scooped or poured by hand, but the management of these substances is frequently required in intermediate or large-scale processes.

Cross-contamination must be avoided while transferring materials for many products using a system. Every material handling system needs to deliver the exact amount of the ingredient to the desired location. Vacuum loading systems, measuring pumps, and screw feed systems are more advanced techniques for handling materials.

In the granulation vessel, a dry blend should occur. A larger batch can be dried and blended before being separated into several pieces for granulation.

There shouldn't be any lumps in any of the ingredients; else, flow issues arise. Before blending, the materials are typically screened or milled to increase the process' dependability and reproducibility. The following tools are used for blending:

Both vertical and horizontal high-intensity mixers, V-blenders, Double cone blenders, Ribbon blenders, Slant cone blenders, Bin blenders, Orbiting Screw Blenders, etc.

Scale up considerations

1. **BLENDING**

To achieve effective medication distribution, powders that will be utilized for encapsulation or that will be granulated before being tableted must be thoroughly blended.

a. Whenever the tablet or capsule is tiny and also the drug concentration is low, inadequate blending could cause drug content uniformity variance.
b. Ingredients ought to be free of lumps to prevent flow issues.

2. **GRANULATIONS**

The most frequently cited justifications for granulation include: - Improving the material's flow characteristics - Increasing the powder's apparent density - Changing its size of particle distribution - making AIP uniformly dispersed- Wet-granu lation has traditionally done by: a hea vy-duty planet tary mixer and signs blade-mixer.

Tumble blenders can also be used to create wet granulation devices with chopper blades that rotate quickly. In recent times the usage of multipurpose processors may complete all tasks necessary to develop a completed product. Granulation, including continuous processes for dry mixing, wet granulation, drying, sizing, and lubricating equipment.

GRANULATION ON A FLUIDIZED BED

- Inlet air temperature for the process.
- Air pressure for atomization.
- Air pressure.
- Spray rate for liquid.
- Nozzle placement and the number of spray heads.
- The temperature of the substance exhausts the porosity of the filter.
- Cleaning intervals.
- Intestinal frequency.

3. SLUGGING (DRY GRANULATION)

Due to its poor flow & compression characteristics, the dry powder could not be compacted directly.

Slugs are compressed with a 15-ton tablet press before being broken up by a hammer mill with the right amount of particle size distribution.

Dry compaction may also be used to granulate powders by passing them between two rollers that are pressed together at a pressure of ten tones every linear inch.

4. WET GRANULATION

The following facilities have to be present to prevent cross contamination during scale-up up and to assist in the cleansing of equipment effectively:

a. The presence of a different room the plus availability of greater space.

b. Granulation must be a unit action.
c. Facilities for washing and drainage are required.
d. Steam, hot, and cold water supply systems are required.
e. Platforms should be made of non-dust or stainless steel materials.
f. Air conditioning is a plus, however, windows need to be screened if it is not present.
g. Utilization of a multipurpose processing system.

5. **DIRECT COMPRESSION METHOD**

When the medicine is dissolved in the granulating solution and introduced during the granulation process, a little amount of a significant active ingredient could be spread in a carrier granulation most efficiently.

6. **DRY COMPACTION**

Pushing powders through two rollers which compact the material at a pressure of up to 10 tones per linear inch can also produce granulation via dry compaction.

To generate a bulk density high enough to permit encapsulation or compression low-density materials requires roller compaction. The densification of aluminum hydroxide is among the best illustrations of this procedure. To create a granulation with the necessary tabulating or encapsulating capabilities, pilot plant staff should assess if the final medication blend or the active component could be processed in this way more effectively than by conventional processing.

7. **DRYING**

The rotating hot air oven, which itself is heated either by steam or electricity, is still the most used conventional technique for drying granulations. The airflow, air temp, and the degree of granulation upon that trays are crucial variables to take into account while scaling up oven drying operations. The drying time will be ineffective if the granulation becomes too deep or dense, and soluble dyes may migrate towards the surface of the granules. Each product and each specific load must have a drying time at a specific temperature and airflow rate. A fluidized bed dryer's scale-up process takes into account factors including ideal loads, rate flows, percentage airflows, inlet air temperatures, and humidity levels.

8. REDUCTION OF PARTICLE SIZE

The first stage in this procedure is to analyze the granulation's particle size distribution to use a series of "stacked" sieves with progressively smaller mesh holes. The dry granulation of production-scale batches can be subjected to particle size reduction by running the entire batch through an oscillating granulator, a hammer miller, a mechanical sieve device, or occasionally, a screening device. The lubricants & glidants are typically directly added to the finished mixture in the laboratory as part of the scaling up of such a mill or sieving operation. This is accomplished because several of these additives, particularly magnesium stearate, have a propensity to clump together when introduced in significant amounts towards the granulation inside a blender.

9. FACILITIES

The following facilitate have to be present to prevent cross contamination during scale-up up and to assist the cleansing of equipment effectively:

a. The presence of a different room plus the availability of greater space. Granulation must be a unit action.
b. Facilities for washing and drainage are required.
c. Steam, hot, and cold water supply systems are required.
d. Platforms should be made of non-dust or stainless steel materials.
e. Air conditioning is a plus, however, windows need to be screened if it is not present.
f. Utilization of a multipurpose processing system.

8. TABLET COMPRESSION

a. The following tasks are carried out by the tablet press during compression:
b. Granulation is used to fill a void in a die that is unfilled.
c. Granulation pre-compression.
d. Granule compression is a process.

e. The tablet is ejected from the die chamber, and the compressed tablet is removed.
f. To identify any potential compression issues, such as clinging towards the punch surfaces, tablet toughness, capping, and weight fluctuation discovered, extended trial runs at pressed speeds are typically used.
g. The capability of the press to engage with granulation is necessary for high-speed tablet compression.
h. The following factors should be taken into account when choosing a high-speed press:

- Granulation feed rate.
- The distribution of particle sizes shouldn't be altered by the delivery system.
- The system should generate static charges and prevent the separation of fine and coarse particles.

i. In the brief time in which the die is moving beneath the feed frame, the die feed system needs to be able to adequately fill the die cavities.
x. It is more challenging to achieve a uniform fill at high press rates for smaller tablets.
xi. A forced die feed system with a range of feeding paddles and speed control capabilities is required for high-speed machines.
l. The tips of the punches typically travel over lower and beneath the top pressure rollers, compressing the granulation in a single motion.
m. As a result, the punches puncture at the die to the specified depth, comp-acting the granu-lation towards the specified distance between the punches' gaps.
xiv. The press's rotational speed and the size of its compression rollers both affect how quickly and how long a press event lasts between occurrences.
xv. The compression force is delivered and released more gradually the larger the compression roller.
xvi. Press speed reduction or the use of a larger compression roller can frequently reduce capping in a formulation.
xvii. The compressed tablets are ejected from the die cavity as the final action.
xviii. When the granulation is compressed to create a tablet, bonds between the materials that are compressible must develop, which causes sticking.

xix. High lubricant concentrations or excessive mixing can make tablets brittle, reduce the powder's wettability, and lengthen the time it takes for them to dissolve.

xx. Designing its die to be 0.001 - 0.005 inches wider just at the upper portion compared to the center to release pressure during ejection is another method for overcoming binding to die walls.

9. **TABLET COATING**

a. Due to new advancements in coating technology (traditional sugar coating pans were replaced with perforated pans or fluidized-bed coating columns), adjustments in safety, and environmental laws, sugar coating has undergone several changes.
b. The transition from aqueous sugar-coated to aqueous coating material has been made possible by the creation of novel polymeric-materials.
c. The tablet should be tough so as to stand up to the tumbling that they experience inside the coating-column.
d. Certain core-material of tablet are hydro-phobic by nature, in that situations, unique formulations of tablet core and/or coating solution may be necessary for film coating with an aqueous system.
e. In a small lab coating pan, a film coating solvent might have been discovered to work with a specific tablet, but on a production scale, it might be completely undesirable.
f. The tablet shouldn't be made with a smooth surface with sharp cutouts to enable efficient coating.
g.

PILOT PLANT DESIGN FOR CAPSULES

Drug components encased in can be hard as well as soft dissolving containers or can be shell made of an appropriate of gelatin in solid dose forms known as ***capsules***. Encapsulation of hard gelatin capsules is done by enhancing good flow properties in which the processed powder mix with the following particle characteristics—particle size distribution, bulk density, and compressibility—is employed to make the capsule. This makes it easier to build compacts that have the proper size and cohesiveness to fit inside capsule shells.

Weight variations in capsules may be caused by inadequate flow properties, an improperly lubricated plug, or a plug that sticks towards the distal plunger interface. Overlay lubrication can cause issues with bioavailability, disintegration, and weight fluctuation. The kind and size of apparatus in use for blending, granulating, drying, sizing, and lubricating have a big impact on the properties of granulation and the completed goods.

HARD GELATIN CAPSULES

COMPOSITION OF SHELL

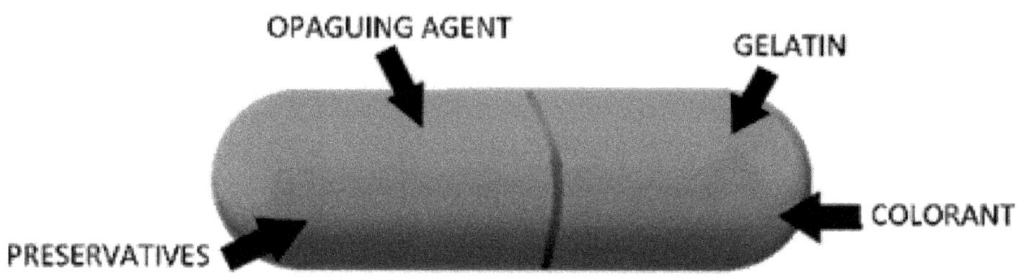

FIG.5: COMPOSITION OF SHELL

1. **Gelatin**: Collagen is hydrolyzed to create it. Gelatin comes in two different basic varieties: Type-A and Type-B. The two varieties can be distinguished from one another by their respective viscosity and film-forming properties, as well as by their iso electric-point. Gelatin made from bone and hog skin is frequently combined to improve shell properties. The bloom strength & viscosity of gelatin are the physicochemical characteristics that shell producers are most interested in.
2. **Colorants**: A variety of insoluble pigments and soluble synthetic dyes, including coal tar dyes, are used. Colorants aid in patient compliance in addition to helping consumers recognize the product. For instance, lavender has hallucinogenic effects, white has analgesic effects, and orange or yellow has stimulant and antidepressant properties.
3. **Opacifying substances**: In the presence of titanium-dioxide, the shell will turn opaque. Opaque capsules could be used to block light or conceal the contents.
4. **Preservatives**: Parabens are frequently chosen when preservatives are used.

SHELL MANUFACTURING

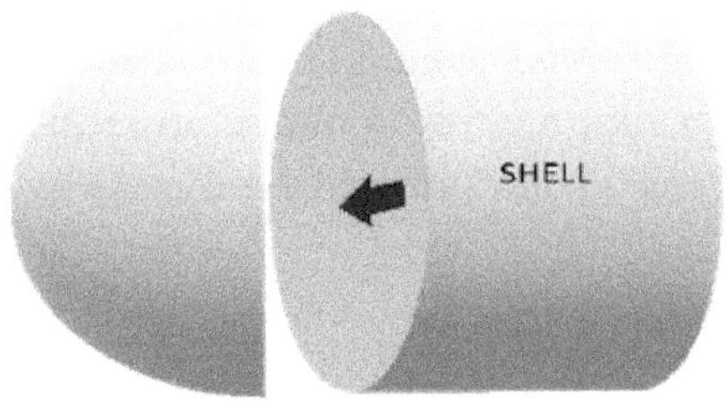

FIG.6: 3-D DEPICTION OF SHELL

STEPS INVOLVED IN CAPSULE MANUFACTURING

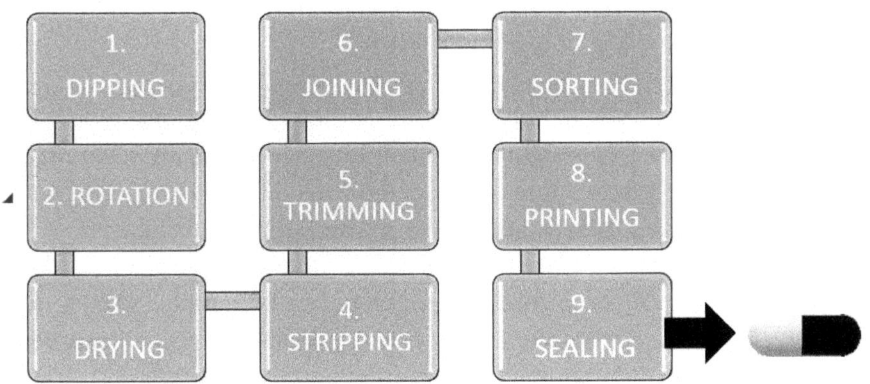

FIG.7: STEPS INVOLVED IN MANUFACTURING OF SHELL

1. **Dipping:**To concurrently produce the caps and bodies, sets of the stainless-steel pins are dipped into the dipping solution. The dipping solution is kept at a temperature of around 50° C within a heated, jacketed dip pan while the pins are kept at room temperature. According to reports, the film's casting process took roughly 12 seconds.

2. **Rotation**: Pins are raised after dipping and turned 2-1/2 times before pointing upward. This rotation aids in even gelatin distribution over the

pins and prevents the development of beads at the ends of the capsules.

3. **Drying**: The gelatin-coated pins are then placed on racks and placed into a set of four drying ovens. Dehumidification is the primary method of drying. To prevent film melting, a temperature increase of just several degrees is acceptable. The films will be too sticky for use after being under-dried.

4. **Stripping**: Cap and body parts of the capsules are separated from the pins by a set of bronze jaws.

5. **Trimming**: The body parts are sent to collectors, where they are securely held, together with the striped cap. Knives are used to cut the shells to the appropriate length as the collectors rotate.

6. **Joining**: The cap and body pieces are pressed together gradually after being concentrically aligned in channels.

7. **Sorting**: The capsules' moisture level as they leave the machine will be between 15 and 18% weight for weight. Inspectors visually scrutinize the scrutinizes they move down a lit conveyor during sorting. Defects are often categorized by type and ability to cause issues during use.

8. **Printing**: Typically, capsules are printed before being filled. Offset rotary presses with throughput rates up to three and a half million capsules per hour are typically used for printing.

9. **Sealing**: In the sealing procedure, capsules are both sealed and somewhat altered. Where the cap overlaps the body, at the capsule's waist, the heat welding process creates an indented ring.

10. **Filling:**One of the following two types of filling methods is frequently employed in capsule filling equipment:

- Zanasi encapsulator: Creates slugs in a catastrophe and has a plun-ger so as eject the capsule-plug.
- Holliger Karg Equipment: Com-pacts are formed at a die plate via tamping- pins.

The scale-up procedure in both of these systems takes into account bulk density, flow property of powder, compressibility, and distribution lubricant. Granules that are too lubricated are to blame for delaying capsule dissolution and disintegration

SOFT GELATIN CAPSULES

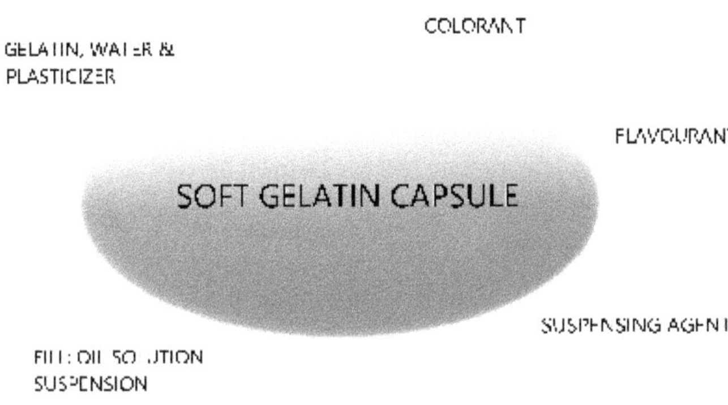

FIG.8: <u>COMPOSITION OF SOFT GELATIN SHELL</u>

<u>COMPOSITION OF SHELL</u>

Soft gelatin shells are made primarily of **gelatin**, much like hard gelatin shells, but the shell has been plasticized.

The "hardness" of the shell is determined by the dry **plasticizer** to dry gelatin ratio, which ranges from 0.3 -1.0 for very-hard to 1.0 - 1.8 for very-soft.

To make the shell more "chewable," up to 5% content of **sugar** may be added.

The completed capsules' residual shell moisture content will be between 6 and 10%.

<u>Manufacturing Processes</u>

1. Plate Process

i. Cover a die plate with plenty of die pockets with the top half of a plasticized gelatin sheet.
ii. Vacuum is applied to pull the sheet into the die pockets.
iii. Stuff the pockets with paste or alcohol.
iv. Refold the gelatin sheet's lower half well over filled pockets.

v. Place the "sandwich" beneath the die press that forms and cuts out the capsules.

2. Rotary Die-Press

i. During this procedure, the outside surfaces of both the two rollers are machined to create the die cavities.
ii. The left side of such capsule is formed by the dies pockets on the left -hand roller, and the right side is formed by the die pockets upon that right- hand roller.
iii. The liquid or paste fill is continuously and simultaneously supplied onto two plasticized gelatin ribbons, which are placed between both the roller of the rotary die mechanism.
iv. As that the die rolls turn, the identical die pockets converge, sealing and cutting out the filled capsules.

3. Accel-Process

i. This procedure uses a measurement roll, a dies-roll, and a sealing roll in general.
ii. The measured dosages are transferred to the gelatin-linked pockets of a die-roll as the measurement roll and die roll revolve.
iii. The second gelatin layer is then applied to create some other halves of the capsule as the filled die continues to rotate and converges with the spinning sealing roll.
iv. The capsules are sealed and cut out by the pressure that is created on between die-roll & sealing -roll.

FORMULATION

Liquid technology is used in the formulation of soft gelatin capsules as opposed to powder technology. Materials are often designed to make the tiniest capsules feasible while maintaining the highest levels of stability, therapeutic efficacy, and production efficiency. Only liquids that won't damage the gelatin walls are allowed. The lipid's pH ranges from 2.5 to 7.5. The inability to fill the emulsion is due to the effect that water release will have on the shell.

There are two primary categories of vehicles utilized in soft gelatin capsules

i. Water soluble, flammable, or most likely more flammable liquids, such as medium-chain triglycerides, vegetable oils, mineral oils, and acetylated glycerides.
ii. Non-volatile liquids that are water miscible have lately gained popularity due to their quick water mixing properties and potential to hasten the dissolving of dissolved or suspended medicines. Examples of these liquids include low molecular weight PEG. All filling fluids must be able to flow by gravity at 35°C or less in temperature. Gelatin films should be sealed between 37°C and 40°C.

PILOT PLANT SCALE-UP CONSIDERATIONS FOR LIQUID ORALS

a. The physical structure of an included medicinal product exhibits Newtonian or Pseudo-plastic flow behavior.
b. At room temperature, it adheres to its container.
c. Liquid dosage forms can take the form of scattered systems or solutions.
d. Two or more phases exist in dispersed systems, with one phase scattered throughout another.
e. A solution is a homogenous mixture of two or more components.

Steps of the liquid manufacturing

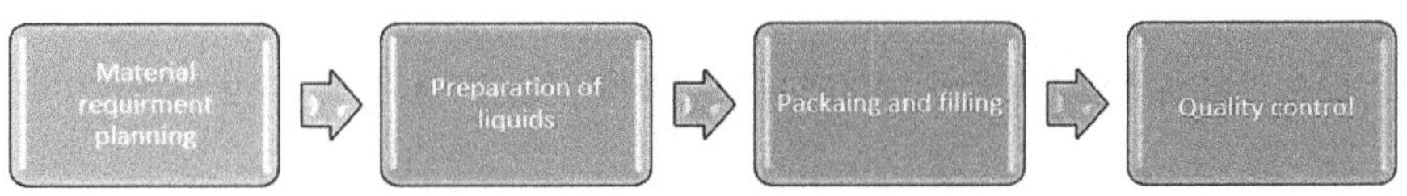

FIG.9 STEPS FOR LIQUID-MANUFACTURING

Critical aspects of liquid manufacturing

a. Physical-Plant
b. Heating, venti-lation, & air-control system.

Effect of prolonged process time at optimal temperatures must be evaluated in the context at the physical & chemical characteristics of ingredients in addition to the product.

SOLUTIONS

The following parameters must be considered when scaling up solutions:

a. Impeller diameter
b. Tank volume (diameter).
c. The number of impellers
d. The type of impeller.
e. The impeller's mixing capability.
f. The impeller's rotational speed.
g. Tank's height filled volume.
h. The no. of baffles.
a. Transfer-mechanism.
j. Clearance that is between the impeller-blades as well as the mixing-tank wall.
k. Filtration-app aratus
ax. Stain less-Steel Passivation

SUSPENSION

The factors to be taken into account when scaling up suspension are;

a. Translator
b. Wetting of the suspending agent
c. Suspending agent addition and dispersion
d. Selection of equipment based on batch size.
e. The amount of time & temperature required to hydrate the suspending agent.
f. Mixing rates
g. Mesh dimension

EMULSION

The following parameters must be addressed while scaling up an emulsion:

a. Homogenizing equipment.
b. The temperature.
c. Mixing apparatus
d. Densities of phases

e. In-process or finished product filters
f. Volumes of each phase
g. Displays, pumps, and filling equipment
h. Viscosities in each phase

PILOT SCALE-UP CONSIDERATION FOR SEMISOLIDS

Semisolid dosage forms, in general, are complicated formulations with complex structural features.

They are frequently made up of two-phases (o/w), out of which one is contin-uous (external) and the other one is dis-persed (internal).

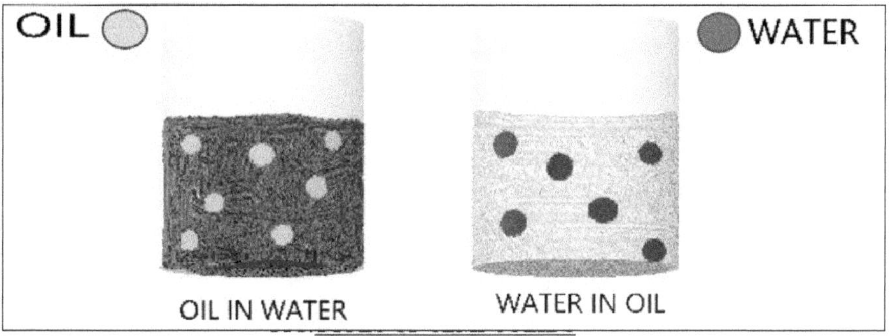

FIG.10: TYPES OF EMULSIONS

The API is frequently absorbed in one phase, however, the medicine is occasionally rarely absolutely soluble within the stem & is spread in 1 or maybe both-phases, resulting in a 3 phase system.

The following parameters must be addressed while scaling up semi-solids:

1. The sequence wherein solutes are supplied to a solvent is frequently unimportant for a genuine solution.
2. However, this cannot be said about dispersed formulations since dispersed matter might diffuse differentially depending on which phases a particulate component is added to.
3. The key moments in a conventional manufacturing process are often the first split of a one-phase system into two phases as well as the stage where the API is introduced.

4. This is especially true for solutes introduced to a formulation at concentrations close to or greater than its solubility anywhere at a temperature at wh ich the output must be exposed.
5. Modifications at the manufacturing technique which occur there-after either phase is likely to be relevant to the end product's attributes.
6. This seems to be especially true for any method aimed at increasing dispersion by lowering droplet or grain size.
7. Process validation studies should especially address the aging of the completed bulk formulation before packaging.

SCALE-UP AND POST-APPROVAL CHANGES (SUPAC):

Scale-up and post-approval changes, such *as those made to medication formulation, batch size, processes, tools, and manufacturing locations, are referred to as* ***SUPAC****.*

SUPAC primarily discusses three stages of change, with each level being assessed using tests for chemistry, manufacturing, and controls, in vitro dissolution, and bioequivalence.

1. Modifications that are unlikely to have any appreciable effects on the performance and quality of the formulation.
2. Modifications that might materially affect the performance and quality of the formulation.
3. Modifications that could significantly affect the performance and quality of the composition.

The following scale-up and post-approval changes (SUPAC) guidance for the industry are combined here, and this advice replaces them: (1) SUPAC-IR/MR Solid &Oral Dosage -Forms, Manufacturing Equipment AddendumSUPAC-SS Non-sterile Semisolid Dosage Forms, Manufacturing Equipment Addendum. It specifies the types of procedures being mentioned while removing the lists of production equipment that were included in both guidance.

The SUPAC: Manufacturing Equipment Amendments draught guidance was released on April 1, 2013. Changes were made in response to comments that were received.

This SUPAC addendum is meant to assist you, the manufacturer, in determining the paperwork you should provide to FDA regarding changes to production equipment. It should be read in conjunction with the SUPAC guidance.

The advice materials provided by FDA, such as this one, do not specify obligations that are enforceable by law. Instead, unless explicit regulatory or legislative requirements are defined guidance should only be considered recommendations. Instead, they express the Agency's conventional understanding of the topic. In Agency guidelines, the word should denote anything that is proposed or advised but not mandated.

LEVEL (L)	CLASSIFICATION	TEST DOCUMENTATION	FILING
LEVEL 1	Quantitatively, a change in the permitted amount of preservative of 10% or less	• Preservative efficacy test at the lowest preservative level specified	• Yearly report
LEVEL 2	10% to 20% shift in the authorized quantity of preservative	• Preservative efficacy test at the lowest preservative level specified	• Changes occurring test supplemented • Yearly report
LEVEL 3	20% modification to the preservative's permitted dosage (including deletion) or the use of a different preservative	• application and compendial specifications • run batch records • Analytical method for identification and test; validation studies; for novel preservative • Test for the efficacy of preservation	• Forgoing approval augmentation • Yearly report

FIG.11: SUPAC LEVEL

ADVANTAGES:

Scale-up runs are easily visible to members of the production and quality control divisions.-

1. The production division has access to supplies of excipients and medications that have been approved by the quality control division in

the more roomy regions available to them.

2. The installation, upkeep, and repair of equipment are possible with the assistance of the engineering department staff.

DISADVANTAGES:

1. There will be less direct communication between the formulator and the production staff in the manufacturing area.
2. Any manufacturing issues will be handled by the staff at the company's pilot facility

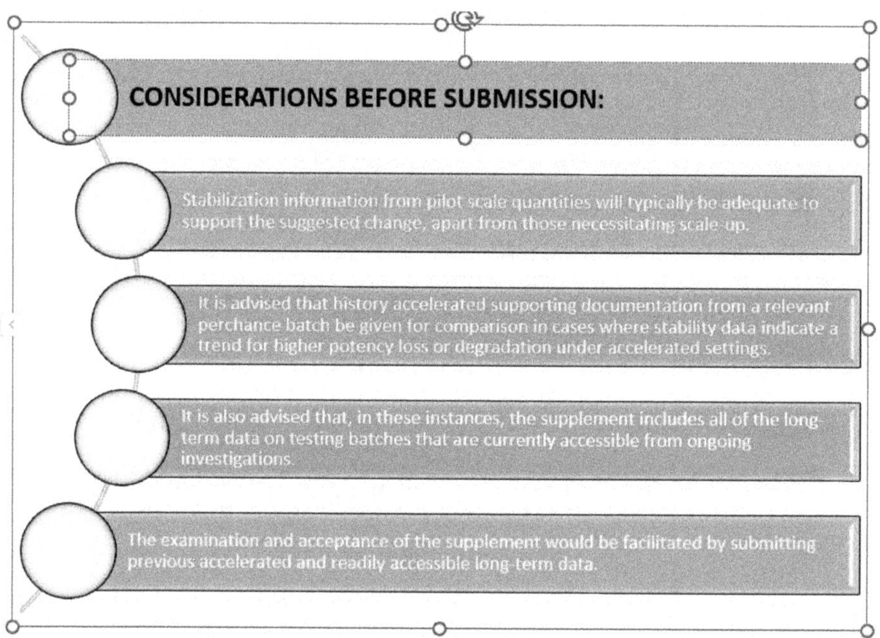

FIG.12: GENERAL CONSIDERATIONS

SCALE-UP AND POST-APPROVAL CHANGES (SUPAC)

Scale-up and post-approval changes, such *as those made to medication formulation, batch size, processes, tools, and manufacturing locations, are referred to as* ***SUPAC***. The following are SUPAC documents or instructions: The FDA publishes a document list to assist applicants with revisions following approval: Documents are separated into SS (Semi-solids), MR (Modified release), and IR (instant release) categories (non-sterile semisolid dosage form)

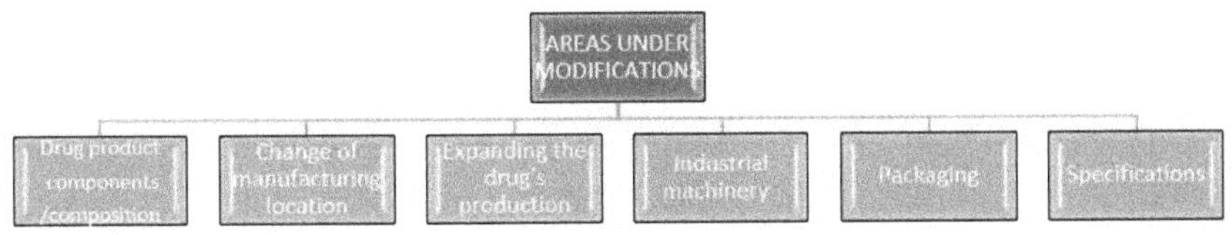

FIG.13: AREAS COVERED UNDER MODIFICATIONS

A) Modifications to the components:

- Section focus at changes to the drug-product's excipients.
- Excipient -SUPAC-M R essential or not for the Modified-drug- release.
- Modifications to excipients that control and prevent release.
- Preservative modifications in formulations for semisolids: -SUPAC-SS
- SUPAC-IR Modifications for solid oral dose formulations with quick release.

B) Modifications to the manufacturing location:

- Relocations of the manufacturing facility, packaging facilities, and/or analytical testing laboratories.
- Avoid include scale-up adjustments, production (including process and/ or equipment) changes, as well as modifications to the components or composition.
- Inspection of current good manufacturing practices(GMP).

CHANGES AT *Level I:*

- CLASSIFICATION: The same machinery, standard operating procedures (SOPs), environmental controls (such as temperature and humidity), and employees are all found in a single facility.

- TEST DOCUMENTATION: Application/compendia requirements for chemistry, solubility, and also in vivo bioequivalence are not required for the test documentation.
- FILING: Annual report documentation filing.

CHANGES AT Level II:

- CLASSIFICATION: No further modifications to classification; same continuous campus; shared employees.
- Testing Records :

1. Requirements for applications and compendia.
2. Revised batch records
3. Address of new site notification

- FILING: Annual report, documentation to be filed.

C) Expanding the drug production:

- The application must include extra information if the size of a batch after approval is changed from the pilot scale biological batch material to bigger or smaller production batches.
- This advice excludes scale-downs below 100,000 dose units.

CHANGES AT$_{\text{Level I}}$:

- CLASSIFICATION: batch size change , up to or a factor of ten times the size-of pilot.
- TESTING DOCU MENTATION: The updated record of batch that meet application compendia criteria stability.
- FILING: Documentation should be filed ANNUALLY.

CHANGES AT Level II:

- Classification: No other alterations, batch size changes greater than ten times the dimensions of pilot
- TEST DOCUMENTATION:

1. Chemistry Documentation Application Release Criteria for Test Documentation.
2. Notification of the modification and batch records that have been modified.
3. Testing for stability: two batches, one testing for long-term stability and the other testing for accelerated stability over three months.
4. Testing for Dissolution Documentation-Case B.
5. There is no in vivo bioequivalence.

- FILING: filing documentation for the annual report and the changes being made add (long-term stability data).

D) Industrial machinery:

Equipment utilized in the manufacturing as well as the process itself may be affected by changes in production.

1. Equipment :

Changes at$_{\text{Level I}}$:

- CLASSIFICATION: Alternative equipment with the same design and operating characteristics as automated equipment.
- TEST DOCUMENTATION: Revised batch records, application requirements, and stability are all included in the test documentation.
- FILING: Pre-approval supplements with the reason for the change and yearly reports are examples of filing documentation (long-term stability data).

CHANGES AT Level II:

- Classification: Switch to machinery with a different design and operating system.
- TEST DOCUMENTATION: Revised batch records, application/ compendia requirements, and stability are all included in the test documentation.

1. Multi-point dissolution spectra in various media using SUPAC IR.
2. Multi-point dissolution patterns in various media using SUPAC-MR.

- FILING: Annual report and adjustments being made supplement filing documentation.

2. Process:

Changes at$_{\text{Level I}}$:

- CLASSIFICATION: Alternative equipment with the same principles and classification as automated equipment
- TEST DOCUMENTATION: Revised batch records, application/ compendia requirements, and stability are all included in the test documentation.
- FILING: Annual report documentation filing.

CHANGES AT Level II:

- Classification: Process adjustments in this group include those that affect mixing durations and operating speed outside the bounds of application and validation.
- TEST DOCUMENTATION:

1. Revised batch records, application/compendia requirements, and stability are all included in the test documentation.
2. Multi-point dissolution profile using SUPAC and IR.
3. Multi-point dissolution rates in various media using SUPAC-MR.
4. SUPAC - SS - Documentation for the in vitro release test.

- FILING: filing documentation for the annual report and the changes being made add.

CHANGES AT Level III:

- CLASSIFICATION: Changes in the type of process employed in the classification
- TEST DOCUMENTATION:

1. Revised batch records, application requirements, stability, bio-study, and IVIVC are all included in the test documentation.
2. Multi-point dissolution profile using SUPAC and IR.

3. Multi-point dissolution spectra in various media using SUPAC-MR.

- FILING: Documentation must be filed including an annual report and a prior approved supplement with reasons.

E. Specifications:

Specifications are the requirements that must be met by a pharmaceutical product to preserve uniformity, repeatability, and quality.

- Unless there is a specific exception from the Regulation guidance materials, such changes necessitate a "Prior Approval Supplement."
- On the following substantial specification changes, except as specified in the SUPAC-IR guidance, prior clearance is required:

1. Relaxing an eligibility requirement
2. Eliminating a specification's entirety.
3. Modifying or implementing a new regulatory analysis method that does not offer the same level of assurance as the one described in the approved application regarding the identity, strength, quality, potency, or strength of the substance being tested.
4. I) 30 days' worth of Changes When there are mild changes to the specifications, such as when a change in the regulatory analytical processes is deemed significant, a supplement must be filed.

II) A modification to the analytical process or the removal of a test for the raw materials utilized in the manufacture of pharmacological substances.

5. Any specifications changes that may have negative side effects on a product but do not compromise its safety and efficacy can be included in an annual report.

F) Packaging:

The life span of the final product can be impacted by the packaging, which is why it is vital. The standards for packaging adjustments have been greatly loosened as a result of the new industry guidance and the stability guidance.

INTRODUCTION TO PLATFORM TECHNOLOGY:

Platform technologies are regarded as an important instrument for increasing quality and efficiency in medicinal product development. The core premise is that using a platform in conjunction with a risk-based approach is the most methodical way to harness existing knowledge for a specific novel chemical. Moreover, such a platform allows for continual improvement by contributing data for each new molecule generated using this approach, boosting the platform's robustness.

The technology provides distinct and distinguishing competitive advantages. Because of its semi-size and adhesive systems for prolonged skin contact, it can considerably improve the bioavailability of complicated substances.

It is also adaptable, containing a diverse variety of active constituents and allowing its systems to be tweaked to attain desired qualities.

Furthermore, the technology is strong and versatile, with significant qualities such as:

1. The active molecule's chemical stability and solubility.
2. High drug levels are possible.
3. Excellent encapsulation efficiency.
4. Created an industrial process with scalability.
5. Technologies that are stable, simple, and solvent-free.
6. Drug reformulation nearing patent expiration.
7. Drug development that was previously thought to be unachievable.
8. New routes of administration for such a platform compounds.

<u>Examples of platform technology:</u>

1. **Nanotechnology**: Using man nanoparticles to deliver medications to types of patient cancer cells, for example, Particles are designed to be drawn to damaged tissues. cells, allowing for direct therapy of those cells.
2. **Technology based on microspheres**: To create distinct formulations for targeted distribution. The goal is to remove the need for repeated doses by using site-specific action. reduce side effects.
3. **Technology for liposomes**: Optimize pharmacokinetics by targeting medications selectively.
4. **Parameters of pharmacological efficacy**, and toxicity reduction, for example, Antibiotic amphotericin B.

5. **Hot melt extrusion technology**: Used to create molecular dispersions with significant advantages over solvent-based methods such as spray drying and co-precipitation.
6. **SR formulations technology**: Used to administer SR (sustained release), modified, and targeted drugs.For example, osmotic controlled release oral delivery system (OROS) tablets.
7. **Technology for multiple unit pellet systems**: Tablets are constructed of numerous particles that break into separate pellets and enable continuous medication release.
8. **Technology for orally disintegrating (OD) formulations**: Used to create OD pills that disintegrate quickly when placed on the tongue, resulting in a speedier onset of action and greater patient comfort and compliance.
9. **Technology for inhalation**: Advantages in the treatment of respiratory disorders Faster action than orally given substance by: Metered dose inhalers, dry powder inhalers, auto-inhalers (steroid and long- ting ß agonist), and nasal sprays are some examples.
10. **Technology based on effervescence**: Effervescent pills are being developed to provide immediate relief as flavor-concealing effects.
11. **Sprinkles**: Specially formulated oral granule formulation for pediatric patients These can be sprinkled on a child's food to make a medicine, such as anti-HIV therapy, more appeal cell-based Stem cell-based products: These can be sprinkled on a child's food to make medicine, such as anti-HIV therapy, and more appealing. Adult mesencthe hymnal cells in the bone marrow are being produced on a large scale for therapeutic uses.
12. **MTCs (magnetic targeted carriers)**: These are micro-particles made up of 75% metallic iron and 25% activated carbon.

CONCLUSION

This report describes solids, liquids, and semisolids scale-up concerns for pilot plants. The pilot plant's major goal is to "Find faults on a small scale and earn a profit on a large scale." The importance of scale-up studies for pilot plants is that they provide a study of the variety of pertinent processing equipment, as well as information on equipment infrastructure and optimization and control of output rate. This provides comprehensive details on the architecture of the pilot plant layout as well as dosage form information, including the varieties of solid, liquid, and semisolid doses as well as the equipment employed in their manufacture.

REFERENCES:

1. Leon Lachman, Herbert A Lieberman, Joseph L Kaniq: The Theory and Practice of Industrial Pharmacy: Section IV: Chapter 23: Pilot Plant Scale-Up Techniques: 3rdedition, published by Varghese Publishing house, 2009; 681-710.
2. James Swarbrick, James C Boylan: Encyclopedia of Pharmaceutical Technology: Pilot Plant Design, Volume 12 New York, 2001; 171-186.
3. Leon Lachman, Herbert A. Lieberman, Joseph B. Schwartz: Pharmaceutical dosage forms: Tablets. Volume 3. second edition. 303-365.
4. Johnny P. Sitompul, Hyung Woo Lee1, York Chan Kim & Matthew W. Chang A: Scaling up Synthesis from Laboratory Scale to Pilot Scale and to near Commercial Scalefor Paste-Glue Production J. of Eng. and Tech. Sci. 2013; 45(1): 9-24.
5. Joseph W. Zawistowski, A.I.A. and Joseph D. Rago, P.E. Pilot Plant Scale-Up Facilities:Establishing the Basis for a Design, 24 J. of pharm. eng. july/ august. 1994; 24-32.
6. KamyaChaudhary, A.C.Rana, Rajni Bala, Nimrata Seth, review: scale up process of tablet production: a prospective discussion, Int. J. of Pharm. and Bio. Sci. 2012; 2(3):223-239.
7. Lippincott Williams and Wilkins, Remington, “the science and practice of pharmacy”,21stedition, 2008; 900-901.
8. Mike , Techceuticals, solution for pharma nutra manufacturers since 1989™?, march 9th, 2009.
9. Faurea P, York RC, Process Control and Scale Up of Pharmaceutical Wet Granulation Process: a review, European Journal of Pharmaceutics and Biopharmaceutics,52,2001,269-277.
10. lsevier, Identifying fluid bed parameters affecting product variability, Anil Menon ,Narinder Dhodi, William Mandella, SibuChakrabarti, International Journal of Pharmaceutics, volume 140, issue 2, 30 august, pages 92-102.
11. Vyas SP, Khar RK. Controlled Drug Delivery:Concepts and Advances. Ist ed. vallabhprakashan,2002, 156 - 189.
12. Shargel L, Yu ABC. Modified release drug products.In: Applied Biopharmaceutics and Pharmacokinetics.4th ed. McGraw Hill.1999; 169 -171.

13. Ratner BD, Kwok C. Characterization of delivery systems, surface analysis and controlled release systems. In: Encyclopaedia of Controlled Drug Delivery, Vol - I. Published by John Wiley & sons.1999; 349 - 362.
14. Nandita GD, Sudip KD. Controlled - release of oral dosage forms, Formulation, Fill and Finish 2003, 10 -16.
15. Malamataris S, Karidas T, Goidas P. Effect of particle size and sorbed moisture on the compression behaviour of some hydroxypropyl methylcellulose (HPMC) polymers, Int J Pharm 1994, 103, 205 - 215.
16. Gohel MC, Parikh RK, Padshala MN, Jena GD. Formulation and optimization of directly compressible isoniazid modified release matrix tablet, Int J Pharm Sci 2007, 640 - 644.
17. Levina M, Palmer F, Rajabi - Siahboomi A. Investigation of directly compressible metformineHCl 500 mg extended release formulation based on hypromellose, Controlled Release Society Annual Meeting 2005, 1 - 3.
18. Jonathan, Bouffard, "Drug Development and Industrial Pharmacy, Influence of Process Variable and Physicochemical Properties on the Granulation Mechanism of Mannitol in a Fluid Bed Top Spray Granulator", 2005,

CHAPTER II

UNIT 2 Technology Development and Transfer

At the end of the chapter, student will understand and gain knowledge about :

Technology development and transfer

WHO guidelines for Technology Transfer(TT): Terminology, Technology transfer protocol, Quality risk management, Transfer from R & D to production (Process, packaging and cleaning), Granularity of TT Process (API, excipients, finished products, packaging materials) Documentation, Premises and equipments, qualification and validation, quality control, analytical method transfer, Approved regulatory bodies and agencies, Commercialization - practical aspects and problems (case studies), TT agencies in India - APCTD, NRDC, TIFAC, BCIL, TBSE / SIDBI; TT related documentation - confidentiality agreement, licensing, MoUs, legal issues

WHO Guidelines for Technology Transfer

These guiding principles for the transfer of technology are meant to act as a framework rather than as rigorous, rigid instructions that can be applied in any situation. According to the mission of the WHO, emphasis has been made on the quality components. In Technology Transfer (TT), existing knowledge, facilities, or capacities are better exploited to meet public and private demands. Basic science research and foundational discoveries are converted into useful and commercially viable applications and products. A logical process that manages the transfer of any technique along with its documentation and professional experience between development and manufacture or between manufacture sites is referred to as a "transfer of technology." There is a methodical process that must be followed in order to transfer to the proper, accountable, and authorized party the documented knowledge and expertise acquired during development and/or commercialization.

Technology transfer includes both the documentation transfer and the receiving unit's (RU) ability to successfully implement the key components of the transferred technology, as determined by all parties and any applicable regulatory bodies.

Technology transfer involves three elements

1. A technical resource (e.g., laboratory)
2. A user (e.g., small business)
3. An interface connecting the two

When referring to the procedures required for successfully moving from medication discovery to product development to clinical trials to full-scale commercialization, the pharmaceutical industry uses the term TT. It is the procedure through which a technology developer makes its technology available to a business partner who will use it.

Technology transfer (TT) is the exchange of knowledge and technical know-how as well as tangible objects and equipment and encompasses a variety of official and informal interactions between technology developers and information seekers.

Purpose of Technology Transfer

By increasing the application of laboratory technology and resources to corporate and public demands and opportunities, technology transfer aims to boost the economy. Successful knowledge transfer initiatives lead to product enhancement, service efficiencies, improved manufacturing processes, cooperative development to address needs of the public and private sectors, and the development of significant new goods for the global market.

Established Technology and Emerging Technology

An established technology: It is one for which cost, and performance data are easily accessible. A technology is only regarded as established once it has been utilized extensively and the outcomes have been thoroughly recorded.

Emerging technology: An innovative technology that is presently being bench-scale evaluated, which involves evaluating a scaled-down version of the technology in a lab.

Technology Transfer Types

Technology transfer can be divided into two categories: vertical and horizontal

Vertical Technology: The technology transfer from fundamental research to applied research, from applied research to development, and from development to production is referred to as vertical technology transfer.

Horizontal technology: It is the movement and use of technology from one place or organization to another, from one business to another, or from one setting with equipment to another.

Advantages of Technology Transfer (TT)

- To clarify the information required to transfer existing product technology between different manufacturing facilities.
- TT develops the market by locating emerging business prospects.
- The processing and evaluation of patent applications, technology commercialization, licensing, and the protection of intellectual property resulting from research effort are all made easier by TT operations.
- By organizing the diverse information gathered during R&D, to clarify the knowledge required to transfer technology from R&D to actual manufacturing.
- TT enables creation of new jobs and financial profit to the employees, researchers, and overall society.
- All of this helps to increase the knowledge and competitiveness of technology providers, start-ups, and innovations, which finally leads to the business arc being widened and the focus being shifted to the technologies and systems to service other fields.
- TT offers economic advantages that increase productivity and effectiveness, market share, and profits.

Disadvantages of Technology Transfer (TT)

The biggest drawback of technology transfer is the financial or commercial risk. Litigation over licensing, patent rights, and other international concerns, such as intellectual property rights, may also result.

Objectives of Technology Transfer (TT)

The two primary components of TT, creativity, and innovation, have the following goals:

- To provide direction and assistance in matters of intellectual property to businesses and inventors.
- To create a venue where entrepreneurs and inventors can meet and trade names and contact information.
- To give students a "hands-on" learning opportunity where they can practice dealing with "real-world" aspects of practicing intellectual property law.
- To spread knowledge about intellectual property and how important it is in the current

information age.

Steps involved in technology transfer:

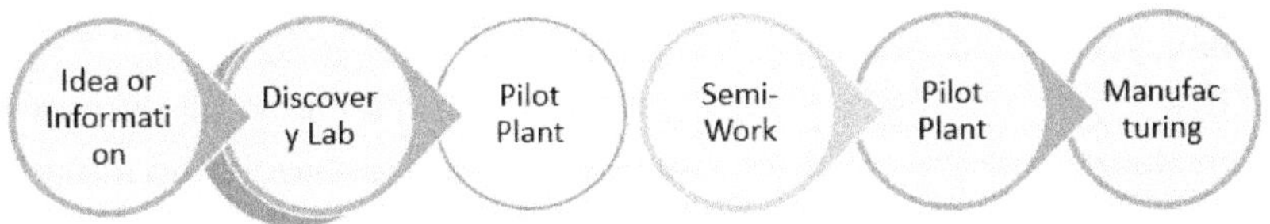

Figure 1: Steps in Technology Transfer (TT)

WHO Guidelines on Technology Transfer

Pharmaceutical firms' constantly evolving business plans increasingly call for intra- and inter-company transfers of technology for needs like the demand for more capacity, the relocation of activities, or consolidations and mergers. At some point during the life cycle of most products, from development, scale-up, manufacturing, production, and launch, to the post-approval phase, processes are transferred to an alternative site.

Guidelines on Technology Transfer have been released by the World Health Organization (WHO) in recognition of the importance of pharmaceutical production on a worldwide scale. Below is a quick summary of the WHO Guidelines on 1Ey Transfer (TT) in Pharmaceutical Manufacturing.

The WHO's technology transfer guidelines are designed to provide a flexible framework with a quality-focused approach. The term "technology transfer" refers to the transfer of documents as well as the receiving unit's ability to successfully carry out the crucial component of technology transfer, to the satisfaction of all parties and any relevant regulatory bodies. In order to satisfy the relevant regulatory body, WHO guidelines provide guidance and general information on the activities required to perform a successful intra- or inter site transfer of technology. The recommendations made in these guidelines are applicable to all dosage forms, although they must be modified individually according to the principles of risk management, for instance, in the case of sterile goods and metered-dose aerosols. The WHO Guidelines are helpful when producing particular pharmaceutical goods. The regulations will be used in the production of active pharmaceutical ingredients (APIs), bulk materials, finished pharmaceutical products (FPPs), and/or analytical testing.

The following areas at the SU and the RU are covered by the Guidelines:

- Transfer of development and manufacturing (processing, packaging, and cleaning),
- Analytical methodologies transfer for QA and QC skills
- Evaluation and instruction, coordinating and overseeing the transfer,
- Evaluation of the facilities and equipment, validation, qualification, and documentation.

Principles of Technology Transfer (TT)

1. It is necessary to adhere to the following guidelines and specifications for the technology transfer to be successful:
2. The planning process should include the project's quality-related components and be built around the management and quality principles. Any lack of openness could result in a less successful transfer of technology.
3. Any successful technology transfer must result in reliable information that gives the recipient party all the details they need to know about the process and related assays. Facilities and equipment should function in accordance with similar operational principles, and the capabilities of the SU and the RU should be comparable but not necessarily identical.
4. Along with meticulous front-end planning and administration, TT calls for assigning employees to particular project components by the project manager. Prior to the process, analytical tests must be transferred. At the receiving site, small-scale verification should be carried out. This demonstrates that the information exchange was successful and enables the recipient party to move on with greater independence.
5. If necessary, a thorough technical gap analysis between the SU and RU should be conducted, including technical risk assessment and potential regulatory gaps.
6. The project plan should cover the quality-related parts of the project, and it should be built on the concepts of quality risk management to identify all potential hazards and develop a strategy for mitigating them. Before transferring technology, a thorough analysis of the technological and regulatory gaps between the sending location and the receiving site should be conducted. Change control procedures should be used to

handle technology transfer.

The following elements must be considered when assessing technological and regulatory gaps:

1. During the risk assessment, it is important to consider the equipment equivalence between the transmitting site and the receiving site in terms of capacity and operating principle. A suitable risk mitigation plan, such as process optimization, critical control parameter identification and process validation with receiving site equipment, batch S1Ze determination based on the equipment capacity, etc., should be proposed if the equipment at both sites differs in terms of capacity and operating principle.
2. Prior to the transfer of technology, the manufacturing formula, method of manufacture, bulk specification, and final goods specification should be frozen and approved.
3. It is important to confirm the comparability of the area classifications for the sending site and the receiving site. Classification of both manufacturing locations should be same and evaluated in accordance with predetermined standards, as well as requirements for raw materials and finished goods like relative humidity, temperature, viable and non-viable counts, differential pressure, etc.
4. Water quality from both the sending site and the receiving site, including raw water, filtered water, water for injection, and pure steam, should be evaluated for its value. There shouldn't be a microbial limit higher than completed items. Before using a product, it is important to qualify it against set specifications.
5. Engineering runs prior to GMP should always be carried out. Reviewing the entire TT project and identifying GMP success and failure is necessary. The team should not be disbanded until success has been established.

Various terms used in the process of technology transfer (TT)

Acceptance criteria: Measurable conditions under which they will be deemed acceptable.

Active pharmaceutical ingredient (API): Any material or combination of substances that is intended for use in the production of a pharmaceutical dosage form and that, when so used, becomes an active ingredient of that pharmaceutical dosage form is known as an active pharmaceutical ingredient (AP). These compounds are designed to provide pharmacological action or other direct effects in the diagnosis, treatment, mitigation, or prevention of disease, or to alter the structure and function of the body.

Bracketing: A method of carrying out an experiment that solely examines the extremes of, instance, dosage strength. The design anticipates that any samples between the extremes will be representational of the extremes.

Change control: It is a formal process by which knowledgeable representatives of the relevant disciplines examine proposed or current changes that could have an impact on a status that has been validated.

Conflict of interest (CO): It is a situation in which a person's professional decisions or actions at his organization (such as a university) may be influenced by factors of personal gain, typically of a financial nature, as a result of interests outside his/her organization's (such as a university's) responsibilities.

Commercialization: The method used to introduce a new good or service to the general public.

Copyright: Authors of "original works of authorship," such as literary, dramatic, musical, artistic, and some other intellectual works, are protected by copyright laws, both formally and informally.

Intellectual property: A phrase that is frequently used to refer broadly to property rights developed via the creative and/or intellectual efforts of a creator and that are typically protectable under patent, trade secret, copyright, and other laws.

Invention: A brand-new and practical method, apparatus, product, or material composition, or a new and practical enhancement of one of these.

Inventor: One who, individually or in collaboration with others, contributes to the invention's conceptualization.

Innovation: It is a new idea, method, or apparatus.

Critical control point (CCP): A stage at which control can be applied and is necessary to prevent or eliminate a pharmaceutical quality hazard or to reduce it to a tolerable level is known as a critical control point (CCP).

Commissioning: The process of configuring, adjusting, and testing a piece of machinery or a system to make sure it satisfies all the criteria given in the user requirement specification. and cation, as well as capacities that the designer or developer has specified. Qualification and validation come before commissioning.

Design qualification (DO): Documented proof that the premises, supporting systems, utilities, equipment, and processes were created in compliance with the standards of good manufacturing practices (GMP).

Design space: The multidimensional interplay and combination of input variables (such as material qualities) and process parameters that have been shown to offer assurance of quality.

Drug master file (DMF): A facility, procedure, or product's specific information provided to the regulatory body in order to be included in the application for marketing authorization is known as the detailed master file (DMF).

Finished pharmaceutical product (FPP): Pharmaceutical product that has completed all steps of production, including labelling and final packaging in its container. One or more APIs could be present in an FPP.

Good manufacturing practices (GMP): This aspect of quality control ensures that pharmaceutical goods are regularly manufactured and controlled to the quality standards necessary for their intended use as well as specified by the marketing authorisation.

Gap analysis: Finding essential components of a process that are present at SU but absent at RU.

In- process control (IPC): Checks made during production to monitor and, if necessary, modify the process to ensure that the product complies with its specifications. In-process control also includes the monitoring of the environment or equipment.

Installation qualification (IQ): The act of testing to determine whether the installations (such as machines, measuring devices, utilities, and production locations) utilized in a manufacturing process are correctly chosen, installed, and functionally in line with established standards.

Material transfer agreement (MTA): A legal agreement that controls the exchange of tangible research materials between two organizations when the receiver plans to utilize the resources for their own study.

Operational qualification (OQ): It is the documented confirmation that a system or subsystem operates as intended throughout all expected operating ranges.

Performance qualification (PO): Documented confirmation that a piece of equipment or a system consistently produces results within predetermined limits and standards over an extended period of time.

Process verification: A high level of assurance that a particular process will consistently produce a product that matches its planned standards and quality features is provided by documented evidence.

Quality control (OC): Quality control refers to all actions taken to ensure that raw materials, intermediates, packaging materials, and finished pharmaceutical products meet established specifications for identity, strength, purity, and other characteristics. These actions include specification setting, sampling, testing, and analytical clearance.

Quality policy: An organization's overarching goals and direction in relation to quality.

Quality assurance (QA): It is a broad notion that includes everything that can individually or collectively affect a product's quality. It is the entirety of the plans put in place to guarantee that pharmaceutical items are of the calibre needed for their intended purpose.

Quality risk management (QRM): It is a systematic procedure for the evaluation, control, communication, and review of risks to the product's quality throughout its life cycle.

Receiving unit (RU): The departments within an organization to which a specified good, service, or method is to be transmitted.

Sending unit (SU): The related disciplines from which it is expected that a given product, process, or method will be transferred.

Standard operating procedure (SOP): An authorized procedure providing instructions for carrying out authored written tasks that must be specific to a given product or material (for example, equipment, operation, maintenance, and cleaning, validation cleaning premises and environmental control, sampling, and inspection).

Start-up company: An entrepreneurial endeavour that aims to fill a market demand by creating or providing an innovative good, process, or service. It is often a recently established, quickly expanding company. A start-up is typically a firm that aims to quickly create a scalable business model, such as a small corporation, a partnership, or an organization.

Trademark: A trademark is a term, name, symbol, or other design that is used to identify the source of goods and set them apart from those of other people in commerce.

Technology transfer (TT): It is the process of giving someone else the official right to utilize and profit from new inventions and discoveries made via scientific study. Copyrights, parental controls, and licensing innovations are all forms of protection.

Technology transfer report: A formal overview of a specific technology transfer effort that includes the methods, standards of acceptance, outcomes, and conclusions.

Validation: The process of demonstrating and documenting that any procedure or method actually and consistently produces the desired results is known as validation.

Validation master plan (VMP): A validation master plan, often known as a "VMP," specifies the areas and systems that must be validated, describes the qualifying criteria, and offers a written roadmap for obtaining and maintaining a qualified facility.

Validation report (VR): A validation report is a written document that compiles data, analysis, and recommendations for process or equipment improvement from a validation program that has been completed.

Technology Transfer Protocol-

The transfer of technology from R&D to manufacturing sites and, from one manufacturing site to another manufacturing site are the subjects of the protocol. This strategy can be used to move technology from the development stage to a manufacturing site or from one manufacturing site to another.

- The protocol addresses both
- The transfer of technology from R&D to manufacturing sites.
- The transfer of technology from one manufacturing site to another.

This strategy can be used to move technology from the development stage to a manufacturing site or from one manufacturing site to another.

The following are the key elements of Technology Transfer Protocol (both transmitting site and receiving site):

1. If any differences are found, a comparison of the material, method, and equipment with the specifics of the action plan is made.
2. Experimental design and acceptance criteria for analytical method.
3. The transitional stages, with proof that each important stage has been successfully completed before the next begins.
4. Identification of critical control points
5. Training and skill development
6. Protocol approval

7. Project schedule for qualification batches, process validation batches, and trial batches (optimization batches).

By working together, the workers from the sending site and the receiving site should carry out any procedure for optimization, process validation, packaging validation, analytical h transfer, or method validation in order to comprehend the process and acquire process-based knowledge. The sending site and receiving site stakeholders should develop a final technology transfer summary report with a conclusion and agree on it in the end. Any change during the technology transfer process should be handled through change control process followed by risk assessment.

Stages of TT includes

1. Scope
2. Objective
3. key personnel and their responsibilities, parallel comparison materials, methods, and equipment.
4. Transfer stages with documented evidence that each critical stage has been satisfactorily accomplished before the next commences.
5. Identification of critical points
6. Experimental design and acceptance criteria for analytical methods
7. Information on trial production batches, qualification batches and process validation
8. Change control for any process deviations encountered
9. Assessment of end-product
10. arrangements for preserving samples of active components, intermediate products, and completed products, as well as information on reference substances when appropriate, and
11. A conclusion that includes project manager warning.

The process and its supporting functions should be validated, and SU should supply the relevant documentation. Typically, an existing process is transferred, and the necessary paperwork is already there. Before transfer, SU or a third party should evaluate the RU's suitability and level of preparedness with regard to the facility, equipment, and support services (such as purchasing and inventory control mechanisms, quality control procedures, documentation, computer validation, site validation, equipment qualification, water for pharmaceutical production, and waste management).

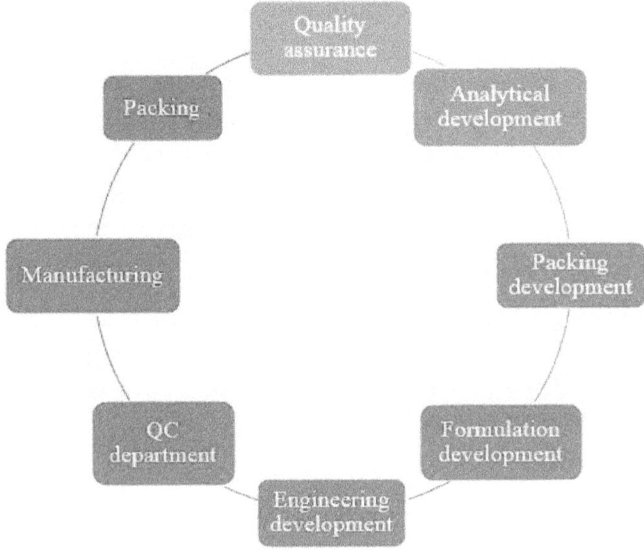

Figure 2: Technology Transfer (TT) Process

Transfer from R&D to Production-

In pharmaceutical industry, TT refers to process of successful progress from drug discovery to drug development, clinical trials, and finally full-scale commercialization.

The anticipated production capacity should be supported by the RU. either continuous production or single-batch manufacturing, for instance. The level and depth of information to be transferred should be considered in order to enable production and any future process development and optimization at the RU as envisioned by the transfer project plan. The technical know-how, site technology, and site capabilities for the RU should all be considered. Any process robustness issues should be identified beforehand by the SU so that the RU can decide.

TT team includes:

R&D process technologist- Focus on transfer activities, collects documents and internal assessment.

Quality assurance representative- Reviews documentation to determine compliance with market authorization, reviews analytical methods with QC to determine capability of equipment's.

Engineering representative- Reviews equipment requirement, initiates required engineering modifications and reviews preventive measures and calibration impact.

Production representative- Reviews process instruction to confirm capacity and capability, verify safety implications, considers impacts on standard operating procedure (SOPs).

Quality control representative- Reviews analytical requirements, availability of equipment's.

Stages of TT involved in R&D-

- Development of technology by R&D.
- Technology transfer from R&D to production.
- Optimization and production.
- Technology transfer documentation.

Success of TT depends upon:

1. Open and direct communication between all team members.
2. The sending and receiving unit must be equally involved.
3. Team work

TT in R&D consists of:

- Production master formula
- Manufacturing and dispensing instructions
- Analytical method
- Cleaning instructions and previous cleaning validation.
- Active specification and source
- Packaging instructions
- Process deviation file, analytical deviation file
- Specimen manufacturing batch record

Granularity of TT process-

The level of detail considered in a model or decision-making process is referred to as "granularity." It describes the degree to which a system is made up of easily identifiable parts. The level of detail increases with increased granularity. In most cases, granularity is used to describe the scope or amount of detail in a set of data.

Granularity of TT Process comprises of following consideration:

Active Pharmaceutical Ingredient:

API/Excipient Synthesis API finish Drug products Direct delivery to patient Printing Capsule filling Reconstitution Innovative devices Primary Manufacturing (Bulk) Secondary Manufacturing the Sending Unit (SU) should offer the Receiving Unit (RU) with the open (applicant's) part of the API master file (APIMF) or Drug Master File (DMF) or Active Substance Master File (ASMF) and any important supplement data on an API suitable for manufacturing pharmaceutical products.

Examples of data which may be provided

- Manufacturer and related supply chain.
- Stage of the API to be transferred
- Flow chart of synthesis pathway, including entry point for raw materials, important steps, process control and intermediates.
- Definitive physical form of API and polymorphic and solvate form.
- Solubility profile
- pH in solution
- Partition coefficient and its determination procedure
- Intrinsic dissolution rate and its determination procedure
- Partition coefficient and its determination procedure
- Water content and determination of hygroscopicity
- Microbial consideration
- Specifications and validations

Excipients:

The final product is influenced by the excipients to be used. The Sending Unit (SU) should provide the Receiving Unit (RU) with their specifications and key functional features (RU)

Ideal excipient qualities include:

1. Reliable and repeatable.
2. No unintended medication interactions.
3. Inert pharmacologically.
4. The functionality you want.
5. Coast successfully.

Example of data which may be provided are:

- Manufacturer and related supply chain.
- Explanation of functionality, with validation for addition of any antioxidant, preservative, or any excipient.
- Solubility profile.
- Intrinsic dissolution rate and its determination procedure.
- Partition coefficient and its determination procedure.
- Bulk physical characteristic.
- Compaction properties.
- Melting point and pH range.
- Particle size and distribution and its determination procedure.
- Specific density.
- Ionic strength.

Finished products:

The Sending Unit (SU) should give a through description of the product, its qualitative and quantitative composition, physical description, manufacturing method, in-process quality control, control procedure and specifications, packaging constituents and configurations and safety and handling requirements. The sending Unit (SU) should offer data on the history of process development that may be needed to all the receiving unit (RU) to make any additional development or process enhancement after transfer.

Packing materials:

The transfer of packing materials should adhere to the same protocol as the transfer of manufacturing. The specifications for an appropriate container or closure systems, as well as any significant supplemental information on design, packing, processing, or labelling requirements, and tamper-proof required by the packing components to qualify at RU, are included in the data of packaging to be transferred from SU to RU. The RU shall undertake appropriate research for the initial qualification of the packing components based on the data. Packaging is deemed suitable if it provides enough protection, safety, compatibility, and performance.

Cleaning:

If the factory is processing many items, pharmaceutical products and APIs may come into contact with one another during the manufacturing process.

Appropriate cleaning processes are crucial to reducing the risk of contamination and cross-contamination, operator exposure, and environmental consequences.

Site-specific cleaning processes and their validation.

Additional information should be provided, as appropriate and where available, e.g.: cleaning validation reports (chemical and microbiological); Ø Information on cleaning agents used (efficacy, evidence that they do not interfere with analytical testing for residues of APIs, removal of residual cleaning agents); Recovery studies to validate the sampling methodology.

Documentation:

- The most important step in the TT process. Important documentation cited in WHO recommendations Depending on the timing, amendments should be made
- Documentation essential for technology transfer:
- SOPs; TOT protocol; training procedure Process validation protocol and report, validation protocol for cleaning, qualification procedure, and protocol for the transfer of analytical methods location and equipment.
- The following two conditions must be met in order to manufacture pharmaceutical products: Locations Instruments Setting Information on design, layout, construction, and services is sent to RU by SU (temperature, water, power etc).

Information on Process and Finished Pharmaceutical Products:

The SU should give a thorough description of the product, detailing its physical characteristics, manufacturing process, in-process controls, control method, specifications, packaging elements and configurations, as well as any safety and handling considerations. In order to allow the RU to carry out any additional development and/or process optimization following a successful transfer, the SU should also give the following details on the history of the process development.

- Information on clinical development, such as details on the purpose of the synthesis, the choice of route and form, the technology used, the tools available, the clinical trials, and the makeup of the final product.
- Information on full-scale development activities, including the quantity and use of manufactured batches, as well as deviation and change control.
- Information on full-scale development operations, including how many manufactured batches are used, their quantity, and their purpose, as well

as deviation and change control.

- Information or a report on full-scale development operations, including the quantity and use of manufactured batches, as well as deviation and change control reports that led to the current manufacturing process
- Information about problem investigations and their conclusions.

Implementation of Processing, Packaging and Cleaning Systems:

Before beginning formal validation, trial batch(es) are typically created to verify process capability. Process validation and cleaning validation can be carried out once process capability has been established at the RU, ensuring that the product, process, or technique there complies with predefined and justified specifications.

Qualification and Validation:

Documentation of qualification and validation is required. The level of qualification and/or validation that needs to be done should be decided upon using the fundamentals of risk management.

Premises and Equipment-

Premises:

The SU should provide information to the RU on the layout, construction of building and services including ventilation, heating, air conditioning (HVAC), temperature, relative humidity, power, water, and compressed air), which have an impact on the product, process, or method to be transferred.

The SU should provide relevant information on health and environmental issues such as:

- Health and safety requirements to minimize operator exposure e.g., atmospheric contaminants or dust, xenobiotics).
- Risk associated with manufacturing processes e.g., reactive chemical hazards, fire, and explosion risks.
- Emergency plannings e.g., is case of spillage, gas or dust release, fire explosion, water run-off.
- Identification of waste streams and provisions for re-use, recycling, and disposal.

Equipment:

The SU should provide a list of equipment associated with the use of manufacturing, filling, packing or control of the product.

Documentation included in this are-

- Manuals
- Drawings
- Maintenance logs
- Calibration logs

Procedures such as equipment set-up, operation, cleaning, maintenance, calibration, and storage.

The RU should review the information provided by SU together with its own inventory list including the qualification status (IQ, OQ, PQ) of all equipment and systems, and perform a side-by-side comparison of equipment at the two sites in the term of their functionality and qualification status.

The RU should perform gas analysis to identify the requirement for adaptation of existing equipment, or new equipment, or change in process, to enable the RU to reproduce the process being transferred. GMP requirements should be satisfied.

Factors to be compared includes:

- Minimum and maximum capacity
- Critical operating parameters
- Critical equipment components
- Material for construction
- Critical quality attributes
- Range for intended use

Quality control: Analytical Method Transfer

Transfer of analytical methods should accommodate all the analytical testing required to demonstrate compliance with the product to be transferred with the registered specifications. Analytical methods used to test pharmaceutical products, starting materials, packaging components and cleaning samples. Process validation samples may be tested at the RU, the SU. A protocol defining the steps should be prepared for transfer of analytical methods. These analytical methods should include description of objectives, scopes and responsibilities of the SU and RU.

The SU responsibilities for the transfer of analytical methods are to:

- Provide method specific training for analysis and other quality control staff.
- Assist is analysis of QC testing results.
- Define experimental design, sampling methods and acceptance criteria.
- Provide details of the equipment's used.
- Provide approved procedures used in testing.
- Review and approve transfer reports.

The RU responsibilities:

- Review analytical methods provided by the SU and formally agree on acceptance criteria before execution of the transfer protocol.
- Provide a documentation system capable of recording receipt and testing of samples to the required specifications using approved test methods, and of reporting, recording and collating data and update of status.
- Ensure that necessary equipment for QC is available and qualified at the RU site. The equipment used by the RU during the analytical transfer should meet appropriate specifications to ensure the requirements of the method or specification are met.
- Ensure that adequately trained staff and personnel are in place for analytical testing.

- Generate and obtain approval of transfer process.
- Execute the transfer protocol.
- Perform the appropriate level of validation to support the implementation of the methods.

APPROVED REGULATORY BODIES AND AGENCIES:

The process of drug discovery and development on the critical thinking and perseverance of researchers and clinicians who work for years to bring medicines to patients. However, the initial idea wouldn`t become a medicine if it weren`t for the role of regulatory agencies, which help to assure the rigor of the data to support the approval of a potential medicine.

Governments of different countries endeavour to promote and commercialise Technology Transfer through various means and regulate the same. The exact regulatory agency that takes part in this process varies by country. Individual countries exert the right to evaluate the quality, safety and efficacy of new medicines for their citizens. Generally, a ministry of health or government department of health oversees this function. This department often includes specific regulatory agencies. Such as the FDA, or Food and Drug Administration in the US, responsible for pharmaceutical product oversight. In some global areas, these bodies operate on a regional basis, while in many countries, they operate at a national level.

While there are several differences between countries in the details of regulatory approval, the very basic approach is similar from place to place.

The overall goal is similar for each of the countries – to evaluate the quality, safety, efficacy, and timely availability of new medicines to their citizens. However, the approaches for exactly how, and at what scale, that review occurs can be very different from country to country.

Approval timelines for potential new medicine globally can vary widely, from less than 1 month to several years. Priority review procedures do not officially exist in most countries globally. However, depending on the product (e.g., new therapy for life- threatening diseases, infectious diseases and cancer) companies can negotiate accelerated review timelines with many regulatory agencies on a case-by-case basis.

Most of the regulatory authorities make a reference to the concept or technology transfer in their respective regulatory frameworks. European Union`s Guidelines for Good Manufacturing Practice for Medicinal Products for Human and Veterinary use makes multiple referenes to technology transfer. It states that GMPs apply to technology – transfer activities.

FDA has addressed the issue of technology transfer in their Guidance titled Contract Manufacturing Arrangement for Drugs: Quality Agreements.

Some of the international regulatory agencies and organizations, which play essential role in all aspects of pharmaceutical regulations related to drug product registration, manufacturing , distribution , price control, marketing, research and development and intellectual property protection etc, include : (i) World Health Organization (WHO), (ii) Pan American Health Organization (PAHO) , (iii) International Conference on Harmonization (ICH) , (v) World Intellectual Property Organization (WIPO).

Some of the regulatory agencies and organizations established in respective countries include (i) USFDA(USA), (ii) MHRA (UK) , (iii) TGA (Australia) , (iv) CDSCO (India) , (v) HEALTH CANADA (CANADA) , (vi) MCC (South Africa) , (vii) ANVISA (Brazil), (vii) EMEA (European Union) , (ix) SFDA (China), (x) NAFDAC (Nigeria), (xi) MEDSAFE (New

Zealand), (xii) MHLW (Japan), (xiii) MCAZ (Zimbabwe), (xiv) SWISSMEDIC (Switzerland), (xv) KFDA (Korea), and (xvi) MoH (Sri Lanka).

Technology Transfer and Commercialization (TTC):

The pace and effectiveness of such a process has a substantial impact on the contribution of the respective public investments to economic development of the country and calls for awareness regarding (i) its processes and the key factors involved, (i) the conditions that enable such processes, (iii) the factors that affect such demand, and (iv) the rationales and means of policy intervention.

By now, we clearly understand that 'Technology Transfer' (TT) refers to the movement of know-how, skills, technical knowledge, procedures methods, expertise or technology from one organizational setting to another. For example, transfer of such assets from research institutions and universities to firms or government institutions, generating economic value and industry development.

The increasing attention to the process through which ideas and knowledge are transferred from public research organization (PROs) to the marketplace is the realization of the relevance of innovation for economic growth and competitiveness across the globe.

Technology commercialization refers to the valorisations of research and intellectual assets by industry, or the process of taking an idea to market and creating financial value. It is also defined as the process of converting ideas into businesses, and consequentially, jobs.

TTC can generate important benefits for economic development. These benefits are realized through industry-science collaboration and technology transactions that can range from simple technical consultancy all the way to licensing of intellectual property. By improving the process of knowledge transfer, countries can foster innovation and thereby raise productivity, create better job opportunities, and address social challenges.

The transfer of technology from the academic to the private sector can happen in several ways: (i) through the formation of start-up companies (ii) through sponsored research agreements with private industry and (iii) through publication of innovations.

Process and Actors: Technology transfer and commercialization (TTC) occur through formal and informal channels:

Formal channels include training and education, hiring students and researchers from universities and PROs (Public research organizations sharing of equipment and instruments, technology services and consultancy, sponsored research and R& D collaboration, and other mechanisms.

Informal channels include the transfer of knowledge through publications, conferences, and informal exchanges between scientists. TTC do not evolve naturally and linearly from research and discovery of scientific solutions.

TTC are executed through the active participation and support of various-individuals and organizations, which undertake activities that evolve around the production of knowledge, the provision of essential supporting services, training , market research and intermediation. Such actions have a common goal i.e. adding value to the process and supporting the technology transfer and commercialization.

Factors affecting demand for TTC: TT forms a path of using and exploiting existing and new knowledge for product development and commercial purposes. TT channels and mechanisms vary across economic and institutional contexts as these determine the availability of knowledge stock, facilitate (or inhibit) the organization, capabilities and interactions of key actors and influence technological choices. These factors impact the demand for commerciality exploitable knowledge and are critical points of consideration for policy makers.

Policy Intervention in TTC

The potential benefits stemming from TT to different users and its commercialization justify the policy makers interest in planning supporting instruments aimed at alleviating institutional gaps, mismatches and barriers.

Strategic interventions and support for TTC appear to be necessary in following areas:

a. Improving institutions, regulations and practices to foster an efficient and more dynamic intellectual property (IP) management system;
b. Developing strategic partnerships between the business community and knowledge centers to conduct research applied to key economic areas and improving the performance of the technology institutes;
c. Accelerating the formation rate of new technology firms and the necessary financing mechanisms;
d. Developing the requisite skills and competences to support the above;
e. Strengthening technology extension capacities and stimulating its demand;

f. Nurturing universities' third mission of contributing to economic growth ; and
g. Fostering an innovative and entrepreneurial culture.

Governments have been making efforts to widen and improve the use of public research output aid to: (i) ensure a sound policy-making context, (ii) alleviating funding barriers, (iii) Strengthen the links between science and industry, (iv) provide knowledge services, (v) establish a clear regulatory framework, and (vi) foster education. Policy sustainability is critical in this process and the need for a long-term political horizon is essential.

Technology Transfer Performance Indicators:

The commercialization of technology transfer may be assessed through the following Technology Transfer Performance Indicators:

License agreements	• Number of licenses executes. • Number of licenses that included equity. • Number of licenses active on last day of fiscal year. • Number of licenses executed in fiscal year to start-ups.
License income	• Number of licenses yielding income in fiscal year. • Number of licenses yielding running royalties. • Total license income of the institution.
Patent-related activity	• Number of inventions discoloured received. • Total patent applications field in India and aboroad. • Number of patents issued in India and abroad.
Start-up companies	• Number of start-ups during fiscal year that depended on licensing of institution's technology. • Number of start-ups during fiscal year where institutions holds equality. • Level of investments achieved by the aforementioned start-ups.
Licensed technologies, post-licensing activity	• Number of licensed technologies that became available for commercial or consumer use during fiscal year.
Other	• Income from negotiating new research agreements and other non-licensing duties.

**Indicators are best expressed as % of research activities conducted at the knowledge centers in the TTO network.*

Technology Transfer Performance Indicators

Case Studies:

Many research universities across the world offer technology transfer services in a sustainable manner.

University of Minnesota Technology Commercialization facilities the transfer of university technology and ideas to licensee companies both established and start-up – for the development of new products and services that benefits the public good,foster economic growth, and generate revenue to support the university's mission, It also provides a range of support services for entrepreneurial researchers interested in forming a start-up company based on University Minnesota inventions.

The university holds 900patents and 1800 current licenses for medicines and health, biotechnology, chemistry, engineering , agriculture, and other fields important to society and the economy. Since 2006, the university has spun out more than 150 start-up companies.

In financial year 2018,it completed a record number of 230 licenses for technologies and 86 sponsored research agreements.

Two more cases of the University of London and the university Technology Enterprise Network (UTEN) in Portugal are were mentioning.

University of London has large research-intensive colleges -Imperial college and University college-with yearly research budgets exceeding US$150 million and each has its own technology transfer office (TTO). The next tier of colleges in terms of size of research budget-including Kings College and Queen Mary College plus two others-have created an alliance. This alliance offers a full range of TTO services to four colleges, each of whom has a significant research budget but insufficiently strong to sustain a full high-quality service.

University Technology Enterprise Network (UTEN) in Portugal took the process a step further by planning to build an integrated national system of TT offices to support all the country's research universities. The initiative was launches by the Ministry for Higher Education and Science as part of a broader strategy to increase the quality and research orientation of the universities through strategic alliances with prestigious research groups in leading global universities and research centres, especially in the United States. The strategy includes upgrading professional skills and exchange of personnel to achieve international connectivity as well as competence.

University of California, a multi-campus university, also set up its TTO as a centralized structure serving all of its campuses spread throughout the state. Over time, as the demands and business opportunities at the local campuses have increased substantially, many functions have been devolved to the local campuses while the central structure has remained responsible for overall coordination.

In China, selected universities have adjusted their performance evaluation framework to recognize commercialization and technology transfer activities in addition to teaching skills and publications.

Literature alerts: International Journal of Technology Transfer and Commercialisation (LJTTC) provides an authoritative source of information in the field of knowledge and technology transfer and diffusion, as well as commercialization and related disciplines.

Conclusion: Commercialization of any scientific discovery and invention is the ultimate dream of any scientist, which requires a seamless integration of science, engineering and economics. The global status of any country depends on its technological development. It is essential to develop and implement indigenous technologies in the country to realize true and sustainable development. India is an expanding economy and expected hub of pharmaceutical manufacturing industries. Therefore, there is a tremendous potential to develop and commercialize indigenous technologies in India. Research institution, industries and supportive Government policies can play vital role in commercialization of indigenous technologies.

TECHNOLOGY TRANSFER AGENCIES IN INDIA

Technology in India is growing exponentially and has played an important role in all round development and growth of economy to the country. India has preferred a wise mix of original imported technology. Developing countries like India generally do not follow the usual path for development with regard to technologies but use their advantage in the cutting edge technology options. Technology transfer in India is not confined to the pharmaceuticals but is broadly catagorized in other areas too such as agriculture, dairy and other technologies.

Government of India is facilitating technology transfer by opening Technology Transfer Offices (TTO) , Technology parks, Universities and other institutions, which shall act as mechanism for transferring or exporting the research conducted and it's outcome to the desired place Government support is quite encouraging as evident from 'start up' companies.

The following agencies have made significant contributions in terms of technology transfer:

TIFAC (Technology Information, Forecasting and Assessment Council)

Need for undertaking technology forecasting and assessment studies on a systematic and continuing basis was highlighted in the Government of India's Technology policy statement of 1983. It further made mandatory, for the Ministries and Agencies with large investments or large volume of production to provide a technology forecast covering their requirements over a 10 year or longer period and for evolving suitable strategies for developed based on priorities.

TIFAC is an autonomous organization set up in 1988 under the Department of science & Technology trajectories, and support innovation by networked actions in select areas of national importance. TIFAC continues to strive for technology development in the country by leveraging technology innovation through sustained and concerted programmes in close association with industry and academia.

TIFAC embarked upon the major task of formulating a Technology Vision for the country in various emerging technology areas. In more than 25years of its service to the nation, it has delivered number of technology assessment and foresight reports.

Technology Vision 2035 aims to make the entire population of India fully aware of basic hygiene practices and ensure sanitation through appropriate and affordable technological interventions. Four ambitious components are:

Foresight: TIFAC has helped in the process of developing ones for other important industrial segments.

Innovation: TIFAC works very closely with the Industry, academia and public research laboratories aimed to address specific sectoral problems.

Patent Facilitation: Patent facilitation center provides patent facilities for scientists and technologies in the country for Indian and foreign patents on a sustained basis.

Linkages: TIFAC is currently the National Member Organization (NMO) of the international Institute of Applied systems Analysis (IIASA)

Recognizing the need for quality manpower and therefore, quality higher education for transformation of the country from a developing one to a developed one, a mission embedded in Technology Vision 2020 was launched by TIFAC on October 4,2000. First ever concerted effort in the area of higher education, the Mission REACH (Relevance & Excellence in achieving new heights in educational institutions), has endeavoured to put in place, a saturated mechanism that can produce world- class manpower of high relevance to Indian industries/ Organizations. The mission aims to create a constellation of world-class Centers targeting excellence in areas of relevance to Indian industries and in turn, the society. COREs (Centre of Relevance and Excellence) created by Mission are luminous examples of real working industry- academia linkage, a concept which the country has been thirsting for.

Under the TIFAC CORE initiative in Herbal Drugs, JSS college of Pharmacy, Ootakmund has developed and transferred:

a. HAPNEZ., a Polyherbal syrup formulations (natural appetizer) for children developed and commercialized through technology transfer by M/ S Tablets India Ltd, Chennai.
b. (b) NSF-3, a Polyherbal tablets formulation for sleep developed and commercialized through technology transfer by M/S Tablets India Ltd, Chennai.

Delhi College of Engineering is one of the centers in the area of Fiber Optics and Optical Communications. The activities of this TIFAC-CORE at DTU is supported by TIFAC/ DST, Govt. Of NCT of Delhi and partners from industries under Mission REACH Program, Technology Vision-2020, Govt. Of India.

HR Nahta College of Pharmacy, Mandsaur (Mp) was accorded with status of SIRO (Scientific and Industrial Research Organization) by the Department of scientific and Industrial Research, Ministry of Science & Technology, Government of India for its Technopreneurship program, which is aimed at commercialization of innovative ideas. This recognition has basically come because of the research and industry collaboration mitiatives taken-up by the institution.

The TIFAC CORE program in Pharmacogenomics at Manipal College of Pharmaceutical Sciences envisages the development of personalized medicine.

TIFAC is situated at Department of Science and Technology, 'A' Wing Vishwakarma Bhavan, Shaheed Jeet Singh Marg, New Delhi 110016 , India.

NRDC (Natural Resources Défense Council)

The Natural Resources Défense Council (NRDC) is a United States-based , non-profit international environmental agency, with its headquarters in New York City and offices in Washington, D.C., San Francisco, Los Angeles, New Delhi, Chicago, Bozeman and Beijing Founded in 1970,tge NRDC works to safeguard the earth -it's people, it's plants and animals, the natural systems on which all life depends.

In 2001, NRDC launched the Bio Gems Initiative to mobilize concerned individual in defence of exceptional and imperilled ecosystem. NRDC has published a number of studies on nuclear weapons stockpiles around the world, both as monographs and as individual studies in the Bulletin of the Atomic Scientists. In December 2006, Green Day and NRDC jointly launched a website to raise awareness on the petroleum dependence of the US.

Some of the environmental programs run by NRDC are mentioned below:

a. The nuclear program that opposes nuclear weapons.

(b)The climate and clean Air Program focuses on clean air, global warming, transportation, energy efficiency, renewable energy, and electric-industry restructuring.

(c) The water and oceans program works on issues related to the nation's water quality, fish populations, wetlands and oceans.

(d) The Health Program works on issues involving drinking water, chemical harm to the environment, and other environmental health threats with the goal of reducing the amount of toxins released into the environment.

(e) Save the Bees Initiative appealing to the president to take urgent action necessary to save the bees populations from further decline.

(f) The Land Program works on issues related to national forests, parks, other public lands, and private forest panda, and works to reduce consumption of wood products.

(g) The Urban Program focuses on environmental issues in urban centers and surrounding areas.

(h) The International program works worldwide on rainforests, biodiversity, habitat preservation, oceans, marine life, nuclear weapons and global warming.

BCIL (Biotech Consortium India Limited)

BCIL is a public limited company, promoted by the Department of Biotechnology (DBT), Ministry of Science and Technology, Government of India and All India Financial Institutions for providing the necessary linkages among stakeholders and business support for facilitating accelerated commercialization of Biotechnology. Inaugurated in 1990 by the then Prime Minister of India, BCIL has been actively involved in technology transfer, project consultancy, fund syndication, information dissemination, and manpower training and placement related to biotechnology over the last decade and half. It has assisted hundreds of clients including scientists, technologies, research institutions, universities, entrepreneurs, the corporate sector, national and international organizations, central government, various state governments, banks and financial institutions.

BCIL acts as an interface between technology sources and technology seekers both within and outside the country. By virtue of the network of national and international linkages established by BCIL, it assists in Technology sourcing, marketing tie-ups and identification of joint venture partners.

BCIL executed the License Agreement with National institute of Cholera and Enteric Diseases (NICED) on behalf of ICMR and Hilleman Labs. for transfer of Shigella Vaccine technology developed by lCMR – NICED to MSD Wellcome Trust Hilleman Laboratories Pvt. Ltd., New Delhi for further scaling up and commercialization on April 23,2019.

Shigellosis is an infectious discase, marked by diarrhoea and fever caused by shigella species. The market size for this vaccine is approximately 2.3 billion globally and 19.8 million in India based on the number of children in the age of 0-6. Till date, there is no licensed vaccine for Shigellosis and treatment options are diminishing due to increasing resistance to key antimicrobials. In this scenario, vaccines are the only effective tool to flight against the disease. The shigella vaccine, developed by NICED ICMR is expected to have a huge impact by largely benefiting children living in developing countries.

Small industrial Development Bank of India (SIDIB)

SIDBI is a development financial institution in India, headquartered at Lucknow and having its offices all over the country. Its purpose to provide refinance facilities and short-term lending to industries and serves as the principal financial institution in the Micro, small and Medium Enterprises (MSME) sector. SIDBI also coordinates the functions of institutions engaged in similar activities. It was established on April 2, 1990, through an Act of parliament. SIDBI operates under the Department of Financial Services, Government of India.

SIDBI is one of the four All India Financial Institutions regulated and supervised by the Reserve Bank; other three are EXIM Bank, NABARD and NHB. They play a salutary role in the financial markets through credit extension and refinancing operation activities and cater to the long-term financing needs of the industrial sector.

SIDBI is active in the development of Micro Finance Institutions through SIDBI Foundation for Micro Credit, and assists in extending microfinance through the Micro Finance Institutions (MFI) route. Its promotion and development program focuses on rural enterprises promotion and entrepreneurship development.

It operates a refinance program known as Institutional Finance program. Under this program, SIDBI extends Terms Loan assistance to Banks, Small Finance Banks and Non-Banking Financial Companies. Besides the refinance operations, SIDBI also lends directly to MSMEs.

State Bank of India is the largest individual shareholder of SIDBI with holding of 16.73% shares, followed by Government of India and Life Insurance Corporation of India.

Andhra Pradesh Commercial Tax Department (APCTD)

APCTD is the nodal agency for the administration and collection of various taxes in the state of Andhra Pradesh. This regulatory body is engaged in managing revenue regulation combines with best practises to run a progressive tax administrative system.

The prime focus of APCTD remains on bringing in greater transparency, fairness and firmness to achieve highest tax efficiency through the use of information technology.

ADCTD Started using SAS (Statistical Analysis System) software to detect tax evasion in various forms and arrest the revenue leakages because of fraudulent dealer. Advanced analytics solutions by SAS have helped APCTD pinpoint evaders and uncover hidden links that indicate collusion for all major revenue sources.

SAS links all the data of various dealers in one place. The software examines the data given by a dealer in different formats at different times and highlights discrepancies. There is also a mechanism in place to integrate and analyse the data from other departments like public distribution system to identify possible cases of tax evasion. In the first phase, fraudulent transactions are detected and then the software further helps in identifying the dealer associated with such transactions. using this data, the authorities plan to issue notices, initiate recovery and levy double penalty on the fraudulent dealers.

Tripura Board of Secondary Education (TBSE)

TBSE was established by Tripura Board of Secondary Education Act. The Board started its functioning from the 1st January, 1976. Intervening period was spent in framing Rules and Regulations, Curricula and Syllabi, and such other guidelines which were being necessary for smooth and active conduct of the business of the Board.

Before 1976, all the High and Higher Secondary Schools of Tripura were affiliated under the West Bengal Board of Secondary Education and the students of Tripura had to appear at the School Final and Higher Secondary Examinations conducted by the West Bengal Board of Secondary Education.

It was in 1976 that the Tripura Board of Secondary Education Conducted its first Public Examinations - School Final Examination [old system, Madhyamik Pariksha (Secondary Examination) [new system] and Higher Secondary Examination [old system]. subsequently, Higher secondary (+2 stage) Examination [new system] was introduced in 1978.

With the abolition of old courses, the Tripura Board of secondary Education now conducts two major Public Examinations- Madhyamik Pariksha (Secondary Examination) and Higher Secondary (+2 stage) [both General and Vocation courses] Examination since 1981.

The Board has introduced the Madhyamik Madrassa Education in 2009. The TBSE is one of the few Boards in the country which has introduced centralised Evaluation system its very inception. Technology transfer and its licensing have played a crucial role in all round development and the advent of the technology, which helps in the development of the economy of the country. This ultimately helps in creating the wealth to the country.

LEGAL ISSUES

Many financial aspects and a number of legal issues, including intellectual property issues, are associated with the transfer of technology or commercialization of technology. However, there are certain key elements that almost every technology transfer agreement must have

These key factors are discussed briefly for the purpose of efficient and productive transfer of technology by strengthening the protection of Intellectual Property Rights.

The Dos of TT

At first instance, it is important to decide that the TT agreement is a licensing agreement of intellectual property or just a know-how agreement concerned with the transfer of statutory recognized knowledge or skills. The content of such TT agreement should be determined on the basis of the motive, strategy, capability, and resources of the organization, which wants to draw technology from the licensor. It will act as a guiding factor in determining the secrecy and confidentiality feature of the agreement.

Typically, the content of TT agreement can be divided into three parts:

(i) mode of transfer, (ii) extent of transfer, and (iii) use of technology under certain terms and conditions. The provisions related to all these should be drafted with utmost caution keeping the following heads in mind:

Specifying the Technology Rights and Territory:

It is fundamental to describe the technology and the rights, which are being transferred in

detail whether being in the form of product or service or just technological knowledge. In the case of complex technologies, the specification of the same with the help of drawing blueprints are important and should cover even minute details so that uncertainty on any aspect of the particular technology should not be left unaddressed. Preferably, a separate

schedule including all rights being transferred should be incorporated in the contract and explicit proviso stating what things are excluded. In the same manner, the territorial jurisdiction for commercial exploitation of the subject technology should also be determined so that the licensor of the subject technology does not directly or indirectly become the competitor of the license. In general practice, parties opt for an exclusive licensing agreement for a specified period in which the licensee has to pay royalty.

Future Improvement and Updates:

It is essential to include the proviso in the agreement that will cover rights in future improvement in particular technology. Such proviso will specifically provide that the updated technology is available to the licensor on specified set of consideration or attracts renegotiation of the contract. In case where improvement of technology is a result of the licensor's efforts, such proviso will sort the ownership issue whether the technology is owned jointly or by the licensee alone. In case the licensee has sole ownership over the improved technology, the licensor can implicit a "Grant-Back Clause" in the agreement, which will bind the licensee to give the licensor rights over the improved technology.

Warranty or Indemnity Clauses:

The main objective of the warranty clause is to save parties from any kind of losses incurred by them because of default on the part of other parties. The licensor will expressly indemnify the licensee that the licensed technology provides specific results and the said technology does not violate the rights of any third party. Such express proviso in the contract binds parties to compensate an innocent party suffering losses.

Confidentiality:

Before framing the confidentiality clause, it is crucial to identify confidential information. Such provisions should expressly provide for the standard of responsibility that the licensee should adhere to while handling the confidential data, especially protecting physical files containing confidential information, enter into a non-disclosure agreement with the allies' whether employees or distributors, vendors, etc. The TT agreement should also provide a list of persons to whom disclosure of such confidential information can be made and what will be the security procedures that have to be followed for maintaining secrecy according to industry standards. Breach of confidentiality by any party, will attract indemnity clauses.

Terms:

In general practice, the patented technology is transferred till expiration of statutory period, but in case of sharing of know-how ortechnology for foreign organizations, the Reserve Bank of India has fixed payment of royalty till a period of seven years from commencement of

commercial production or 10 years from the date of agreement, whichever is earlier.

Prerequisite:

The Reserve Bank of India (RBI) and Secretariat for Industrial Assistance are authorities whose prior approval is mandatory and it is also obligatory to include all terms and conditions of the agreement specified by the RBI in its letter of approval in case of Foreign Technology Transfer.

Dont's of Technology Transfer Agreements

Falling short while negotiating a TT agreement may result in inefficient use of transferred technology. Presence of certain provisions Unjustified Obligations: The obligations, especially on the licensee, in any manner which adversely affect productivity, profitability or efficient monopoly over the technology should be avoided. The licensor having monopoly over the technology tries to impose certain restrictions on the licensee like obligating him/her to acquire raw material, source capital goods, etc., from a distributor specified by the licensor, or engaging the specified class of work force to deal with the subject technology indicated by the licensor. All this may disrupt the purpose of transfer of technology, so all those provisions should be avoided while drafting a technology transfer agreement are as follows:

Fixing the price and resale price of the end product manufactured with the use of subject technology.

(a) Limiting the volume and structure of production.

(b) Clauses which obligate the licensee to pay for the patents or for other industrial property even after expiration of its statutory term.

Absolute Right over Future Improvement: The clauses providing absolute ownership to either party over future improvement carried out by the licensee should also be avoided. Such provisions increase the possibility of dispute at a later stage in case of improvement. So, the issue of future improvement should be properly addressed in the agreement and the rights of all the parties to the agreement should be balanced.

Unreasonable Restrictions: Some unreasonable restrictions that parties try to incorporate in the TT agreement, which the opposite party should consider carefully before approving these clauses, are:

(a) Restriction on the export of the licensed product even if it is not hampering the legitimate interest of the licensor.

(b) Restricting use of technology where the technology transfer agreement has expired except where the termination of the agreement took place at an early stage under the reasons specified in the agreement.

(c) In case of non-exclusive technology transfer agreement. restricting the use of competitive technology.

(d) Restricting the research and development programs on the technology transferred.

These are some of the key features that organizations should look forward to while entering into a TT Agreement. Parties to such an agreement are expected to the sufficiently vigilant and shall opt for mutual benefiting terms so that rights and liabilities of the parties can be balanced and adequate protection to technology can be provided. The main motive of TT should be economic growth and overall technological development which may be hampered by the unreasonable restrictions.

CHAPTER III

UNIT 3 Regulatory Affairs & Regulatory Requirements for Drug Approval

At the end of the chapter, student will understand and gain knowledge about :

RECENT ADVANCEMENTS IN REGULATORY REQUIREMENTS FOR DRUG APPROVAL

Regulatory affairs: Introduction, Historical overview of Regulatory Affairs, Regulatory authorities, Role of Regulatory affairs department, Responsibility of Regulatory Affairs Professionals

Regulatory requirements for drug approval: Drug Development Teams, Non-Clinical Drug Development, Pharmacology, Drug Metabolism and Toxicology, General considerations of Investigational New Drug (IND) Application, Investigator's Brochure (IB) and New Drug Application (NDA), Clinical research / BE studies, Clinical Research Protocols, Biostatistics in Pharmaceutical Product Development, Data Presentation for FDA Submissions, Management of Clinical Studies.

ABSTRACT

Currently, different nations must comply to different regulatory guidelines in order to authorize new drugs through marketing authorization applications (MAAs). The most strictly regulated products in the modern era are pharmaceuticals and medical devices. A lot of research must be done in the fields of chemistry, production, controls, preclinical science, and clinical trials in order to produce a novel drug. Nonclinical drug trials should be carried out after a lead molecule has been identified to guarantee efficacy and safety. Clinical trials can then be conducted following the submission of an application to the relevant country's competent body. The competent authority analyses a request for permission to commercialise a drug and grants permission if satisfied that the drug addresses purity, safety, and performance concerns. Once a new drug has been approved, the government should continue to monitor it for negative effects through post-marketing monitoring, or phase IV.

CONTENTS

1. Introduction
2. Regulatory Affairs Profession

    a. Role of Regulatory Affairs Department
    b. Historical Review of Regulatory Affairs
    c. Importance of Regulatory Affairs

3. Regulatory Requirements for Drug Approval
4. Drug Development Teams
5. Non-clinical Drug Development
6. Investigator New Drug Application
7. Investigator's Brochure
8. New Drug Application
9. Clinical Trials

    a. Phases of clinical trials
    b. Management of clinical studies

10. Clinical Research Protocol
11. Bioequivalence Studies
12. Biostatistics in Pharmaceutical Product Development
13. Data Presentation for USFDA Submissions

INTRODUCTION

Regulatory agencies are the agencies/organization which go ahead with the registration of the drug product. If a company wants to sell or manufacture a product they first need to get the product registered with the regulatory authority of that specific country.

They play a significant role in meeting the legal procedure associated with the drug development method. They control all the rules, regulation, issues attached to these rules and control the drug development methodology, licensing part, registration, production, promoting and labelling of the pharmaceutical product.

Most regulated market in the world is United States Department of Health and Human Sciences Food and Drug Administration (USFDA). It looks after the registration of drug products in United States of America.

WORLDWIDE MAJOR REGULATORY AGENCIES

- India: CDSCO (Central Drugs Standard Control Organization)
- USA: USFDA (United States Food and Drugs Administration)
- Canada: Health Canada
- UK: MHRA (Medicines and Healthcare Products Regulatory Agency
- Europe: EMA (European Medicines Agency)
- Japan: PMDA (Pharmaceutical and Medical Devices Agencies)
- Australia: TGA (Therapeutic Goods Administered)

REGULATORY AFFAIRS

Regulatory Affairs is a profession that covers a broad range of specific skills and occupations. It works as a bridging gap between the people who are coordinating with these regulatory agencies for getting the product registered. Until and unless they get the product registered you cannot sell the products. They have a very critical and specific role which is dealing with the government agencies for the registration process of products which may range from drugs, cosmetics, pesticides, agrochemicals, complementary medicines or alternative medicines.

For selling any product into any country we need to abide by the rules and regulations of that country so each and every country has its own regulatory authorities if you want to register and sell a product over there you need to contact the Regulatory authority of that specific country and need to follow the norms, the guidelines, the advisory issues by that regulatory authority. For example, if you want to market a into United States you have to get the product registered from their agency which is the USFDA.

Role of Regulatory Affairs Department

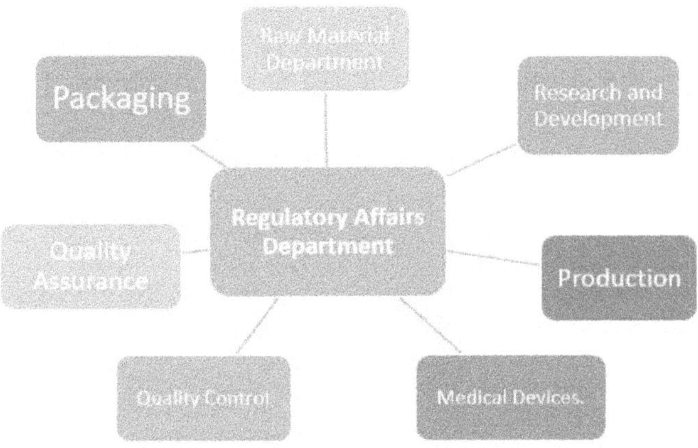

Roles of Regulatory Affairs Department

HISTORY OF REGULATORY AFFAIRS

1. The Pure Food and Drug Act of 1906, the result of 25 years of campaigning, established one of the earliest governments regulating bodies (now known as the FDA), and made it unlawful to sell "adulterated" or "misbranded" food or medicines.

2. The Federal Food, D&C Act of 1938 was passed as a response to the tragedy in which the synthesis of sulphanilamide with a deadly solvent resulted in 107 fatalities. As a result, producers were forced to confirm the safety of their products before marketing.

3. The Kefauver-Harris Drug Amendments of 1962 were passed as a response to the calamity that Thalidomide caused in thousands of European babies. In order to implement better control over drug testing, producers were required to show the efficacy of products before marketing them.

4. The Dalkon Shield, a contraceptive IUD created by the Dalkon Corporation, was discovered to cause severe damage to a disproportionately high proportion of its users, resulting to the 1976 Medical Device Amendments.

5. The 1979 GLP final rule established good laboratory practice for nonclinical laboratory research that supported proposals for research or marketing authorizations for pharmaceuticals for use in both humans and animals, biological medical devices, and biological products.

6. 1991-ICH Guidelines on Safety, Quality, and Efficacy - As the EC, Europe worked to create a single market for pharmaceuticals in the 1980s, it pioneered the harmonisation of regulatory standards. The US, Japan, and Europe were in conversation all at the same time about the potential harmonisation.

IMPORTANCE OF REGULATORY AFFAIRS

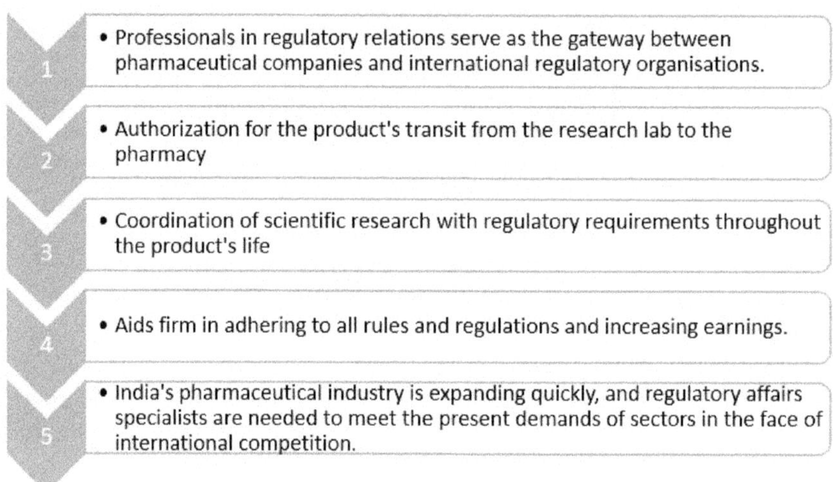

Regulatory requirements drug approval process

The INDA is an application that is to be submitted to the respective regulatory authority of the country for the permission to market a new drug in that country. Once the lead compound molecule is identified for a target disease, it should be optimized for its therapeutic effectiveness. After the discovery of a new drug, pre-clinical trials are conducted on animals such as mice, rat, rabbit, monkeys etc. to ensure safety and efficacy. This is followed by submission of an application to the relevant country's competent authority seeking license for conducting human experiments. Clinical trials are carried out in four important phases to guarantee the efficacy and safety; then the drug dose is advanced into humans. Once clinical trials are conducted successfully sponsor submits MAA, then that is recognized by the appropriate authority; if drug is satisfying the requirements of safety, efficacy and show that its benefits outweigh the risks. In order to get this consent a sponsor should submit a preclinical test data and clinical test data through *NDA* to examine drug information and for knowing explanation of methodologies and the procedure of manufacture adopted.

Following are the different phases of human clinical trials:

I. PHASE I: This phase is called as human pharmacology trial wherein safety and tolerability of new drug is estimated.
II. PHASE II: This phase is called exploratory trial in which effectiveness and short term side effects of new drug are estimated.
III. PHASE III: This phase is called confirmatory trial in which therapeutic benefits of new drug are confirmed.
IV. PHASE IV: This phase is called post marketing trial wherein studies are done after drug approval when the drug is marketed for public use.

Once NDA is submitted to the regulatory agency, it undergoes a technical screening to ensure for sufficiency for data and drug information under each section that justifies the filing of the NDA. Upon reviewing the NDA, any of the three possible actions are taken by agency and are communicated to the sponsor through a letter.

The new drug approval in India is a two phase process –

- Clinical trials
- Marketing authorization of drug

Firstly, non-clinical study of the drugs are finished to ensure its safety and efficacy, then the application for running of human trials is put forward. Then the human Clinical Trials from *Phase I to Phase IV* are conducted. An application is submitted for acceptance of the drug for marketing purpose.

The Regulatory authority reviews the application and accepts the drugs for marketing if the drugs are found effective and safe in humans or the drugs have less adverse effect as compared to its desirable effect. The government monitors the safety and efficacy even after the approval of New Drug, when it is marketed in large populations; like its interaction with other drug which were not seen in a pre-marketing trial and the Adverse Effects are monitored too.

DRUG DEVELOPMENT TEAMS

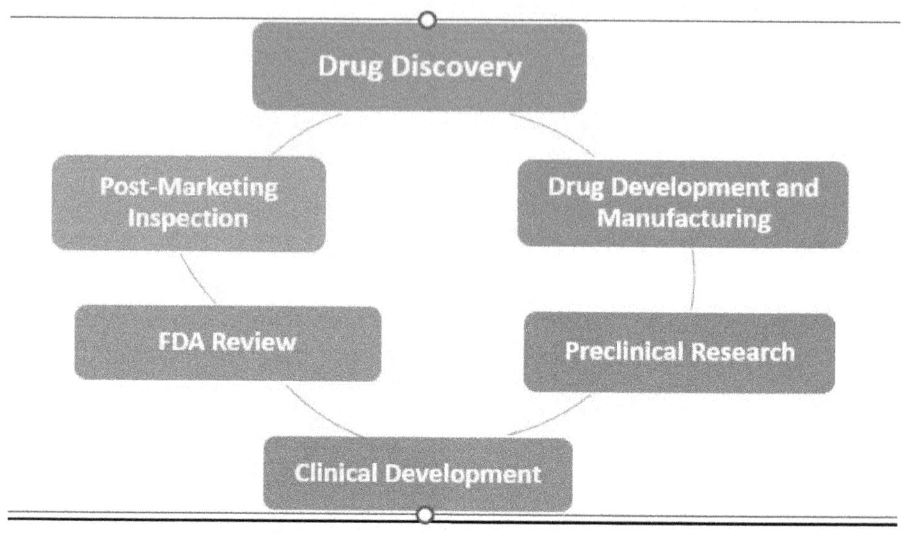

Non-clinical Drug Development

Before proceeding to the clinical phase of development, the non-clinical development phase strives to discover candidate treatments with the highest chances of success, evaluate their toxicity, and provide a strong scientific background.

The research done in the non-clinical development phase includes:

In silico: - this research is carried out using computer simulations. A s in employing data-based methods to anticipate a drug candidate's toxicological profile based on its chemical composition.

In-vitro: - It is carried out by conducting a process in a controlled setting apart from a living entity. Using hepatocyte (liver cells) cultures to study metabolism is one example.

In-vivo: - Experiments are conducted for this research utilizing a complete, living organism, such as an animal, a human, or a plant.

It mainly involves 2 major types of studies

- *Pharmacological Studies*

1. Pharmacokinetic: its primary aim is to determine the ideal dose level and to present data on the dose-effect connection. It addresses the

toxicokinetic and ADME (Absorption, Dissolution, Metabolism, Excretion)

2. Pharmacodynamic: it mainly deals with;

A. Primary- research the drug's physiological effects.
B. Secondary- examine the drug's mechanism of action and any impact of the relevant substance that do not related to the drug's intended therapeutic effect.
C. Safety- it is carried out to find a compound's adverse pharmacodynamic effects on a few physiological functions that might have an effect on human safety.

- *Toxicological Studies*

1. Single-dose: by giving a single, large dose of the test medications to evaluate.
2. Repeated-dose: should be conducted on at least two different species. Examine the effects of daily, low-dose medication administration for 6–9 months.
3. Genotoxicity: it's goal to identify whether the proposed medicine can cause DNA damage, either by making some modifications in nucleotide base sequence or by causing changes in chromosomal structure.
4. Carcinogenicity: A long-term carcinogenicity research is conducted, especially if the medicine is administered for an extended period of time.
5. Development and reproductive toxicity: These investigations assess the potential teratogenicity of the medication candidate, male and female sterility, parturition and the infant, the lactation process, and care of the children.

TYPES OF DRUG REGULATORY APPLICATION

1. Investigational New Drug Application
2. New Drug Application
3. Biologics License Application
4. Abbreviated New Drug Application
5. OVER THE COUNTER (OTC) DRUG APPLICATION

INVESTIGATIONAL NEW DRUG APPLICATION

An Investigational new drug application is emergence in the drug review process. It is a consent to United States FDA seeking consent to, commence the clinical studies of the New pharmaceutical Drug product in United States.

The *IND* is means by which the advocate gets from the USFDA a freedom to Federal law, as the regulatory guidelines require that an investigational drug or biologic should be the subject of *Marketing Authorization Application* before the drug is taken or distributed across state borders. As a sponsor would want to transport the experimental drug to the clinical examiner in many states. To get this freedom the sponsor is required to present enough sufficient data by the INDA reporting the drug safety in humans. There are 2 IND categories:

- *Commercial* - which allows the advocate to gather the data on clinical safety and efficacy required for marketing application in *NDA form.*
- *Research* – which grants permission to sponsor for usage of drug in investigation to get modern empirical knowledge of new drug. Hence, there is no plan to market the drug product.

IND application contains following information :

1. ***Studies on the pharmacology and toxicity of animals*** which gives the information about preclinical research necessary to determine if a medicine is fairly safe for use in human trials.
2. ***Manufacturing information*** including manufacturer information, formation, consistency, and the controls employed in the drug's production. By the help of this knowledge it's ensured that companies can effectively manufacture and give routinely batches of drug in the market.
3. ***Investigator's information*** includes the eligibility of clinical investigators, who look after the administration of candidate drug to study subjects. Its used to evaluate if the investigators are qualified to conduct the clinical trials on humans.
4. ***Clinical protocols*** holds the protocols which regulates if the starting trials may or may not reveal human subjects to unnecessary risks.

INVESTIGATOR'S BROCHURE

IB is a certificate which includes all the clinical and non-clinical data that is needed for the INDA on the investigating drug. The main agenda of this document is to give away the information of the investigators with the other professionals which are in the trials.

It also has the details which helps the investigators to understand about the hypothesis and other main components of protocol like route of administration, method of administration, dose and its frequency and safety monitoring tools. This also gives the vision to help support and understand the clinical management of subjects during the trials being conducted clinically.

IB's general considerations:

1. Description Page – which shall have the sponsors name, specifications of investigating product and its launch date. It is recommended to give a citation to the edition number and date that it replaces, as well as an edition number.
2. Private Statement – which shall have a statement regarding the directing the IB as a protected record for the exclusive knowledge and use of the research team, IRB, and IEC.
3. Investigators brochure information have –

1. The contents list
2. Synopsis
3. Introduction
4. Investigational substance and formulation attributes
5. Non-clinical research

a. Nonclinical pharmacology
b. Animal pharmacokinetics and product metabolism
c. Toxicology

1. Reactions in humans

a. Human pharmacokinetics and product metabolism
b. Effectiveness and safety
c. Marketing knowledge

7. Synopsis of data and advice for investigator

a. Journals
b. Claims
c. Appendices

NEW DRUG APPLICATION

In New Drug Application the pharmaceutical manufacturer or agent asks permission from the USFDA for a license to market a drug for one or more specified implication. An NDA must show the results of clinical trials conducted for which a license is requested in addition to the chemical and pharmacologic description of the drug.

Once the non-clinical studies and clinical studies on human beings have been conducted then comes the stage where the drug sponsor formally proposes that the regulatory body can approve a new pharmaceutical product for sale and marketing which is done through the form number 44.

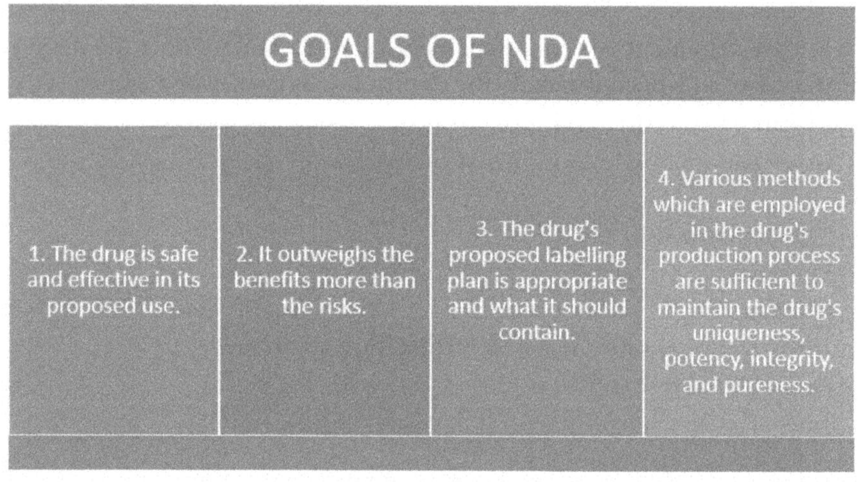

FEW FORMS OF NDA USED-

Form FDA-356h application for marketing a NDA or ANDA or BLA for human use.

Form FDA-3397 if for user fee cover sheet. It is made to determine if a fee is needed for review application tor to know the amount of required fees and to track the user fee.

Form FDA-3331 NDA field report. it is submitted by the drug manufacturer after receiving the information that the drug product labelling mistake or microbial contamination or chemical, physical or other changes during the drug distribution.

NDA general Format

- **Archival copy** – it is a complete copy of NDA which contains the detail that is required under the Application form, Index to the summary section by volume and page number, technical chapters, samples & labelling and the documentation listed under the case report forms.

Applicants may be submit the archival copy on paper or in electronic format except professional labelling which must be submitted to the agency in electronic format.

- **Review copy** – The review copy of the NDA must be provided by the applicant. Each technical component includes things like:

1. Section on chemistry, manufacturing, and controls (CMC)
2. Section on toxicology and nonclinical pharmacology
3. Section on the pharmacokinetics and bioavailability of human drugs
4. The microbiology subsection
5. Section with clinical data
6. The statistical part
7. Pediatric use section,

must always be bound separately and include a version of the application form and summary.

- **Field copy** – copy of the NDA that includes the technical segment CMC, a duplicate of application form, a replica of the summary, and confirmation that the CMC in the field copy is an exact replica of the one contained in the archived and reviewed versions of the NDA are all required submissions from the applicant.
- **Binding folders** – In order to bind the archival, review, and field copies of the NDA, the applicant may acquire enough folders from the FDA.
- **Electronic format submissions** – digital format submissions have to be made in a manner that the FDA can read, process, and keep. FDA will occasionally publish instructions on how to submit the electronic form.

FEW EXAMPLES OF NDA SUBMISSION

New Drug - Fostemsavir

Company – ViiV healthcare

Treatment – HIV Infection

The ViiV Healthcare has submitted NDA for Fostemsavir on 5th Dec.2019 to the USFDA.

New Drug – Paxlovid

Company – Pfizer

Treatment – COVID-19

Pfizer has submitted NDA for Paxlovid on 30th June 2022 to the USFDA.

After submitting NDA the FDA takes 60 days to confirm whether to review the application or dismiss it due to missing information.

After 60 days if all the data is discovered to be adequate, the FDA chooses whether to conduct a conventional or rapid review of the NDA and tell about the application's acceptance and review of their decision in a different correspondence, often known as a 74-day letter. The FDA makes a determination after a normal assessment in ten months.

During this the FDA meets the sponsor at least twice:

- During the conclusion of phase 2 clinical trials
- Before the filing of NDA or pre-NDA meeting.

The analysis committee looks through it and decides whether or not to accept the proposal of application

CLINICAL TRIALS

It is a type of an investigational study that assess new ways to improve the treatment, tests and see their effective outcome on the health of the human. Clinical research is done on subjects to evaluate various medical treatments, including drugs, cells, and other biological products, surgeries, and radiographic methods, gadgets, behavioural therapies, and preventive care.

Before they can begin, they must be approved after thorough design, review, and completion. Clinical trials are accessible to participants of varying ages, even young children.

Process of clinical development

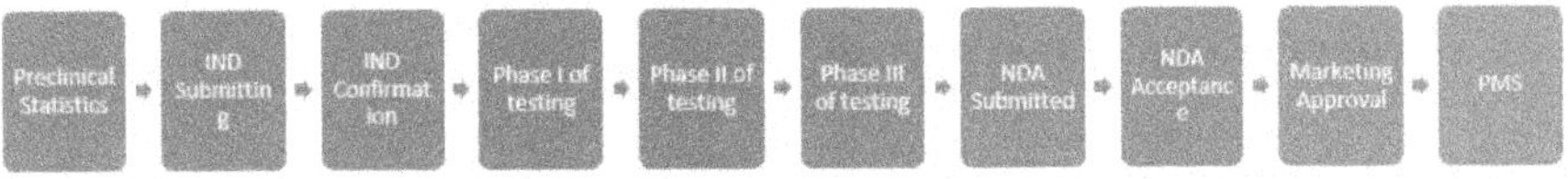

Phases of Clinical Trials

PHASE 1	PHASE 2	PHASE 3	PHASE 4
•Reasearchers test an experimental drug on 20 to 100 healthy volunteers. •Approximately 70% of the drugs move to the next phase. •The primary purpose is to ensure the safety and dosage of drug	•The experimental drug is given to a 100 - 300 people who have disease or condition. •Approximately 33% of the drugs move to the next phase •The primary purpose is to make sure that the side effects are less and to obtain high efficacy.	•The treatment is provided to 500 - 3,000 people needed with the illness/condition •About 25-30% of drugs advance to the next phase. •The primary purpose is to maintain efficacy and monitor the ADR.	•It is onseveral thousand people with the disease or condition. •It is basically up for the post marketing surveillance. •The primary purpose is to maintain the safety and efficacy of the drug.

Management of clinical studies

Clinical data management is the procedure for gathering, purifying, and managing subject data in accordance with legal requirements. Because the information gathered during clinical trials is examined for safety and efficacy, it is a very important step in clinical research. In the pharmaceutical sector, this study serves as the cornerstone for decision-making about product development. The clinical data manager plays a very important role in 3 major earrings these are

- **Study Setup** – includes all the activities before the start of the study. The activities like-

1. Preparing data management plan
2. CRF annotation

3. Database build and design
4. Edit check or Validation rules implementation
5. UAT (User Acceptance Testing)

- **Study Conduct** – starts once the subject enrolment begins or with the first patient first visit. In this the activities like –

  1. Ensuring that data is collected, validated, complete, and consistent.
  2. Central laboratory or third party data transfer
  3. Data Coding
  4. Query management
  5. SAE Reconciliation
  6. Reports generation or Metrics and tracking

- **Study Closeout** – at this step the data is final and ready for statistical analysis ; the activities performed are –

  1. Ensuring all data management activities are complete
  2. Database Lock
  3. Electronic Archival
  4. Database Transfer

Case Report Form

It is a device used to gather all the data from each participant in a clinical research. In order to gather the precise data they need to test their theories and discover the answers to their research questions, the sponsor typically develops or outsources CRF creation.

It is a written, visual, or digital record created to contain all the data needed by the protocol to be submitted to the sponsor on each trial subject.

Types of CRF

1. Traditional Paper CRF – It is a more conventional method of collecting data and is suitable for short studies or those with a broad range of designs.
2. Improvised electronic CRF (eCRF) – eCRFs are considered if studies are large and have same designs.

eCRFs are chosen before paper CRFs as they require less time, which will motivate the sponsor to act out simultaneous broad multicentric research. It is intended to with edit checks in a manner that allows for extremely small errors during data entering. Additionally, the RA are open to applications that utilize use of verified electronic data capture (EDC) methods.

CRF Designing Team

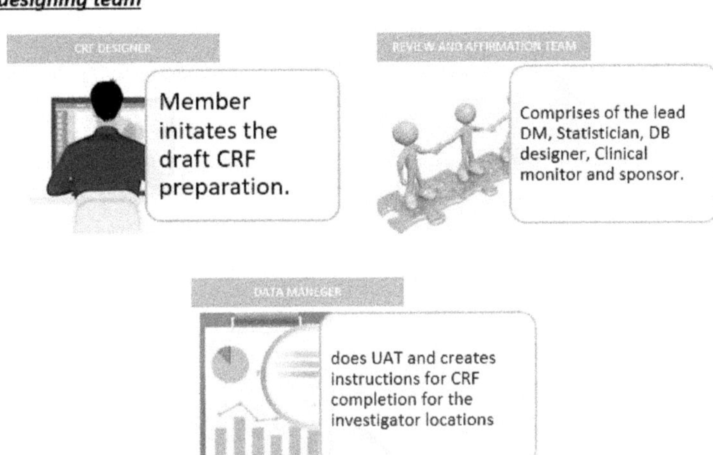

CLINICAL TRIAL PROTOCOLS

It is a legal document which outlines the study plan of the clinical trials in detail yet comprehensive and concise manner. Every clinical investigation starts by growth of the clinical agreement.

A CTP is a report which outlines the setting, thinking, purpose, blueprint, procedure, analytical reflections, and operation of a clinical research project. It contains

v. Study plan on which the clinical trial is based.
v. Types of people that may participate in the trial
v. Schedule of the tests involved
v. Procedures that will be followed throughout the trial
v. Allowed medications as well as prohibited medications
v. Dosages

v. Length of the study

Protocol development: It requires cross functional and collaborative teamwork. The members required in protocol development are :

1. Principle Investigator
2. Biostatistician
3. Medical Monitor
4. Research Scientist
5. Clinical Research Associate
6. Medical Writer

The ICH Good Clinical Practice standards state that the following topics should be covered in a protocol:

- Title
- General Background
- Aim
- Design of the Study
- Subject Selection and Rejection
- Subject Treatment
- Efficacy and Safety Assessments
- Adverse Reactions
- Study Discontinuation
- Statistical Data
- Assurance and Quality Control
- Morals
- Data and Record Management
- Publishing Strategy
- Project Timeline/ Flow diagram
- Citation
- Supplements and Annexes

BIOEQUIVALENCE STUDIES

BE studies provide important information on a up to date product that is planned to be replacement for a certified therapeutic product as a pharmaceutical substitute. They are conducted to:

- Reduce the risk of bio-inequivalence
- Increase the therapeutic effects and decrease the side effects.

Therefore, bioequivalence indicates that when the substance enters the systemic circulation in two or more similar dose forms at the very same rate and with the same extent.; meaning their plasma medication concentration-time profiles won't differ substantially from each other. In order to ensure clinical performances on such drug products Bioequivalence studies are performed.

21 CFR Part 314

Drugs Submitted Under an ANDA: Bioequivalence Investigations considering Pharmacokinetic End - points. FDA has issued a guidance under the same

This suggestion gives guidance to the candidates thinking to include BE information in *Abbreviated New Drug Applications* (ANDA) and *ANDA supplements*.

ABBREIVATED NEW DRUG APPLICATION (ANDA)

A drug product that is equivalent to an innovator pharmac(eutical product is considered a generic drug product. Usually, there is no need for clinical and preclinical safety and effectiveness data. uses of generic drugs considered to be "abbreviated" submissions.

The duration of a generic drug's bloodstream penetration in between 24 and 36 healthy humans is one-way researchers indicate bioequivalence. They can compare the generic medicine's bioavailability, or rate of absorption, to that of the innovator drug using the information provided.

The innovator drug's generic substitute should deliver identical quantity with active components in the same amount of time into the patient's circulation.

Recent Advancements

Major changes in the August 2021 Draft ANDA PK and BE guidance:

- Updated and clarified content on RLD and RS in the Orange Book and references new guidance.
- Broaden the content on the study population with respect to gender(female/male) and age (pediatric and geriatric)
- Revised the proposal on how to evaluate proportional similarity in added dose strengths for the case of modified-release drug products on the basis of mechanism of the release and dissolution profile closeness.

- Included a portion of new dosage form which depends upon systemic Bio-equivalence assessment.
- Attached a new segment of the different routes of administration, containing products administered by *Nasogastric* (NG) tube or *Gastric* (G) tube
- Included a part on the operation of outliners in Appendix A.
- Eradicates the 2013 draught guidance's section on "Orally Administered Medications Meant for Local Action."
- Covers two new appendices (B & C) on reference scaled mean BE studies for medications with a limited therapeutic index and considerable drug variability.

BIOSTATISTICS IN PHARMACEUTICAL PRODUCT DEVELOPMENT

Biostatistics is the utilization of statistics in evolution and usage of the medicinal devices and drugs in humans and in animals. It is a broad chapter of biological sciences which involves various statistical operations such as clinical trials, supervising and designing biomedical tests, and growth of the allied computational data.

Biostatistics is the salient feature in epidemiological investigation, genomics, proteomics, expansion of health schemes, public health management, conformation-based practice in clinical medicine, health economics, and spread of pharmaceutical products.

It mainly comprises of variety of steps like generating thesis; accumulating data; application of statistical study.

BIOSTATICS PLAY A PART IN:

- Recognise and make therapies for diseases and find their side effects
- Know about the illnesses' risk elements
- Create, detect, clarify, analyse and give clinical study findings
- During the stage of planning the experiments, design of experiments (DOE) provides inputs for planning experiments to get the relevant information.
- Play role in all areas of R&D

APPLICATIONS INSIDE PHARMACOLOGY

- A drug is given to humans or animals to evaluate the drug's activity and to determine if the changes it causes are owing to the drug or not.

- To differentiate the action of two separate drugs or two consecutive dosages of similar drug.
- To determine how potent a new medicine is in comparison to an existing one.
- In healthcare –

- Comparing the effectiveness of a specific drug, medication, or mode of treatment
- Finding mutual relationship among two characteristics. Example; tobacco use and oral cancer
- To recognise disease/syndrome symptoms and indications.

Responsibilities of Biostatistician

- Organize the study and formulate the protocols.
- If necessary, create the randomization algorithm.
- Create the plan for the statistical analysis (SAP) programming tables, figures, and listings for the research data based on SAP (TFLs).
- In the clinical study report, give the data and explain how they were interpreted.

DRUG DISCOVERY

Biostatistics new lead in branch of statistics gives the pharmaceutical companies the information that is required to make drug discovery rapidly more efficient and quicker.

For example; antibodies which are an important part of the immune system attach themselves to antigens on the surface of bacteria/virus to label it out as an invader, are being experimented for scope of their usage in the treatment of cancer.

The statistical software made by the Deane group models the antibodies in 3D and anticipate the properties it will have. This program helps the companies to prioritize which antibody they need to further investigate and also helps in designing an entirely latest antibody.

DATA PRESENTATION FOR USFDA SUBMISSION

The FDA can modernise and simplify the review process due to data standards. They also make it possible for analysis tools to be used more consistently, improving the way drug data is viewed and emphasising problem areas.

A standard method of transferring clinical and nonclinical research data between computer programs is described by study data standards.

FDA is implementing new rules for data standards that will be applicable to the majority of study data submitted to the agency's Center for Drug Evaluation and Research (CDER) and Center for Biologics Evaluation and Research (CBER). In order to ensure that data standards are taken into account in the design, conduct, and analysis of studies, they highly advise sponsors and applicants to take into consideration the implementation and usage of research data standards as early as possible in the product development life cycle.

Common Technical Document (CTD) containing 5 modules

CTD is an internationally agreed; well-structured common format for the organization of the technical requirements that is to be submitted to the regulatory authority as an application for the registration of pharmaceuticals for human use in all three ICH regions (Europe, Japan and USA)

CTD is a joint effort of 3 category agencies; EMA, USFDA, MHLW.

It is a set of specifications for a dossier for the registration of medicines.

***Electronic* Common Technical Document (eCTD)**

It is about delivering regulatory filings in an electronic format. The sponsors must adhere to the regulations listed in the FDA Data Standards Catalog;

- studies that commenced after December 17th, 2016 for NDA, BLA, and ANDA
- research on commercial IND conducted after December 17, 2017

FDA verifies sponsors are adhering to the FDA Data Standards Catalog using eCTD validations (1734, 1735, 1736, and 1789).

eCTD's goal and the data needed for the study

- A timely review of study data is essential to the FDA's review procedure. Reviewers, for instance, have 30 days to examine an IND application.
- Sponsors who provide data to the FDA in a trustworthy and usable format increase the efficiency and consistency of review decisions.

CDISC Standards allow the FDA to accelerate up the review procedure:

- Shorten the time reviewers need to find and recognise data collected.
- Lighten the load of Information Requests on Sponsors and Examiners.
- Use data mining and data analysis approaches to assist data-driven decisions.
- Shorten reviewing time by permitting the use of reviewer's tools that are commercially available, such as JReview, JMP Clinical, etc. for automating review analysis.

Technical Rejection Criteria for Research Data specifies the circumstances under which the FDA will not accept submissions containing study data.

- 1734
- 1735
- 1736
- 1789

CDER SUBMISSION PROCESSING

It is a streamline process of determining the submission category

- Process – Determine the submission category relying on the structured facts in the eCTD sequence, which serves as a gateway to the review division.
- Benefit – Reviewers can review submissions sooner, and there is fewer manual data entering.

Challenges to the FDA

The FDA is in the process of automating incoming submissions utilising structured data from the eCTD backbone files and Form 356h in order to efficiently and effectively process the increased volume of submissions and utilise the provided structured eCTD and study data.

The information given in the eCTD backbone files are not always consistent.

CONCLUSION

The protection of public health is the primary objective of regulatory bodies around the world, and they do this by guaranteeing the efficacy and safety of pharmaceutical goods. The advancements in the regulatory affairs are generally triggered by the adverse events due to which the life of the humans is in threat; for e.g.- COVID-19. This report describes the drug regulatory affairs and how are they carried out.

The main aim of drug regulatory agencies is to register a drug for the manufacturing and selling of it. The significance of drug regulatory affairs is in how they help to manage clinical studies in humans, restrict the quantity of drugs that are registered, and keep track of their safety and efficacy. Applications such as INDA, NDA, ANDA, BLA, and others are necessary for the drug approval procedures.

From medication discovery to post-marketing surveillance, there are a few procedures involved in getting a drug approved. Due to recent improvements in the regulatory procedures for drug approval, the public health is better protected from adverse outcomes disaster. Regulatory agencies play a vital role in providing patients with effective healthcare based on their compliance.

CHAPTER IV

UNIT 4 Quality Management Systems

Quality management systems: Quality management & Certifications: Concept of Quality, Total Quality Management, Quality by Design (QbD), Six Sigma concept, Out of Specifications (OOS), Change control, Introduction to ISO 9000 series of quality systems standards, ISO 14000, NABL, GLP

QUALITY MANAGEMENT

Introduction

A management system that is required to produce high-quality products and services and perform the tasks according to the quality specifications is termed as a **Quality Management System (QMS).** The QMSis responsible for proper documentation of policies, processes, and controls for achieving the quality standards and regulatory specifications.

A QMS helps coordinate the functions of an organization to fulfil customer requirements and continuously improve its effectiveness and efficiency.

The QMS integrates all the processes and the process approaches for proper implementation of the programs to identify, measure, control and improve the products and services provided in the market.

The term "Quality Management System" and the acronym "QMS" were given in 1991 by Ken Croucher. He was a British business consultant who worked on the design and implementation of a common model for QMS in the IT industry.

Quality management is the act of supervising all the procedures and processes that must be accomplished to maintain a desired level of excellence. It has four basic elements:

Principles of QMS

Customer Satisfaction
Process Approach
Continuous Improvement
Leadership
Evidence-based decision making
Relationship management

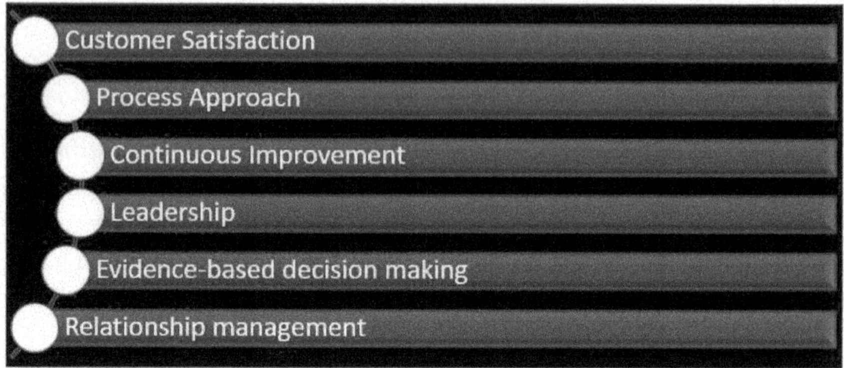

Need of QMS

QMS plays a vital role in the pharmaceutical industry for maintaining the quality and safety of the products and services. The goal of the QMS is to provide best quality products and services along with continuous improvements to meet the regulatory standards and customer needs. Administration of a QMS affects all the functions of the organisation. Some benefits of QMS include the following points:

- Meeting the customer's needs and provide good quality products and services which in turn help the organisation build more customers in the market.
- Fulfilling organisational requirements, which ensures adherence to the rules and requirements of the goods and services in a resource- and cost-effective way, expanding the opportunities for growth and profit.

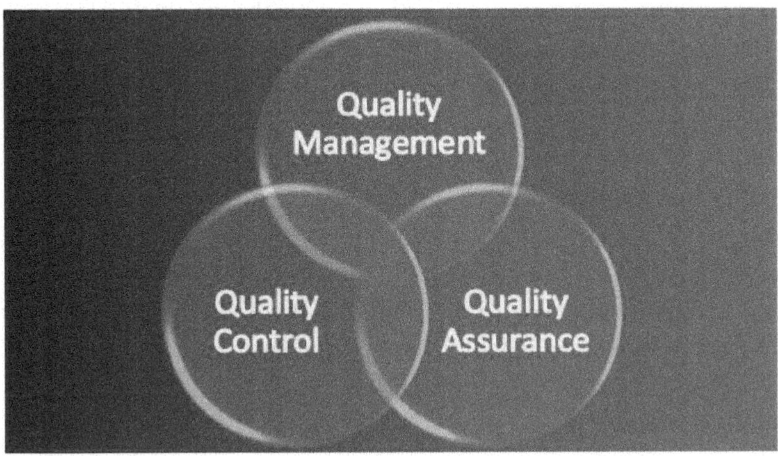

Concept of Quality

The word 'quality' has several definitions. **Quality** can be characterised as meeting the requirements. Quality is the degree to which a product satisfies the necessary requirements. Quality is the comprehensiveness of a product's features and qualities that have an impact on its capacity to meet certain requirements.

Quality in manufacturing can be characterised as a standard of excellence or as the absence of imperfections or contaminants. Quality is accomplished by strict and consistent adherence to certain standards to achieve high-quality products in order to satisfy customer requirements.

Types of Quality

Quality of design and quality of conformance are the two major categories of quality. The first type is related to the design of the product. Improper design of the product has no benefit even if it complies with all the standard specifications.

On the other hand, quality of conformance states the fact that if product does not conform to the design specifications, it will not perform its function in the correct manner.

1. **Quality of Design**

This is related to the characteristic design of the product. The product design should be proper and also comply with the standard specifications. High-quality materials, good and organised processes, high maintenance and high performance are some of the characteristics related to the high-quality product.

1. **Quality of Conformance**

Quality of conformance can be described as a plan, monitor and check strategy in quality management system. It is the ability of a product or service to comply with the product specifications that have been set by the authorities.

Quality Systems

A quality system is formally described as 'the organisational structure, responsibilities, procedures, processes and resources for implementing the management of quality'. A quality system is directly or indirectly responsible for the proper monitoring of the products, procedures, processes and the services within an organisation.

Quality systems have these three basic elements:

1. *Quality Management*
2. *Quality Control*
3. *Quality Assurance*

Quality Management

Quality Management is responsible for the management of the quality of the product and services provided by an organization. Management of an organization is of utmost importance for proper functioning of the organization. It plays a vital role in managing the assets of an organization along with utilising them in an organized manner to reduce the wastage of resources. Proper management increases productivity in all aspects of organization's functions.

Quality Control

QC is a product-based quality system. It is a set of procedures that ensure that the manufactured product meets the specifications. It is responsible for monitoring and maintaining the quality of the manufactured products. Its goal is to detect or identify the defects in the manufactured product.

Quality Assurance

QA is a process-based quality system. Its main function is to maintain the quality of the procedures in the manufacturing process. It identifies the various defects in the processes and also maintains the quality of the processes involved in manufacturing. It ensures that the processes are performed as per the Standard Operating Procedure (SOP). It ensures that the processes comply with the operation specifications. It forms an integral part of the manufacturing operation.

CERTIFICATIONS

Certifications are one of the most important aspects of pharmaceutical industries. Pharmaceutical industry should have a certification from the regulatory bodies to function judiciously. The pharmaceutical sector is heavily regulated and has tight guidelines to follow because pharmaceutical items are essential to health.

The standard quality and effectiveness of pharmaceutical items must be upheld. These items must go through specific controls at every stage of production to guarantee product safety. The International Organization of Standardization (ISO) produces a number of standards for this reason that aid in maintaining the effectiveness, safety, and calibre of pharmaceutical products.

As a result, there has always been a need for ISO certification in the pharmaceutical industry. Additionally, it enables the pharmaceutical firms to outperform their rivals and establish their trust in the market.

Pharmaceutical firms can manage their operations and maintain compliance thanks to ISO certifications. NQA is a recognised certification organisation that has conducted certification audits for numerous pharmaceutical companies. The different certifications for the pharmaceutical industries include the following:

ISO 9001 Standards

The most widely used ISO certification for implementing quality management systems in an enterprise is ISO 9001:2015. It has enormous significance because it ensures the quality, safety, and effectiveness of pharmaceutical products as well as that of the procedures those products go through. It may be applied to any industry and to pharmaceutical firms.

ISO 14001 Standards

Numerous laws have been passed to limit how negatively economic operations affect the environment in response to the growing concern over the state of the environment. The pharmaceutical industry can create and execute an environmental management system with ISO 14001 certification, which will enhance the organization's relationship with the environment and ensure compliance with all applicable environmental regulations.

ISO 45001 Standards

To boost productivity, it's critical to protect the health and safety of your staff. An organisation can develop an Occupational Health and Safety Management System that eliminates any danger to occupational safety by using an ISO 45001 certification.

ISO 50001 Standards

The ISO 50001 certification proves a company's capacity for carbon footprint reduction. The pharmaceutical companies can efficiently use their energy resources and minimise waste with the aid of this certification. These organisations can gain a competitive advantage by raising efficiency and lowering costs.

Need of Certifications

The pharmaceutical business benefits from ISO certifications for pharmaceutical production in the following ways:

Enhancing Organizational Performance

Setting up quality controls will be necessary for ISO certification, which will make your company work more efficiently. The certification procedure offers you the chance to evaluate your company's performance and find ways to increase productivity.

Lower Energy Prices

With ISO 50001 certification, you can work to reduce energy expenses and save money, which your company can use for important activities.

Standards of Quality Assured

Pharmaceutical certifications encourage the application of established best practises, enabling your company to produce safe and efficient pharmaceuticals.

Improved data protection

All businesses are urged to implement thorough information security management systems. Through certifications like ISO 27001, you can reassure your customers and staff that your information is secure.

TOTAL QUALITY MANAGEMENT

Introduction

Known as TQM, Total Quality Management is a management framework used for improving the quality and productivity of the products and services in an organisation. It is a comprehensive approach that works along with the organisation, including all the departments and employees for attaining the required quality and complete customer satisfaction.

Total Quality Management is a continuous process of reducing or eliminating errors in an organisation. The process aims to enhance internal practises continuously in order to increase the quality of an organization's outputs, including its goods and services.

Besides TQM, other acronyms are also used to identify quality-focused management systems. These include QFD (Quality Function Deployment), QIDW (Quality in Daily Work), SQC (Statistical Quality Control), TQC (Total Quality Control), and CQI (Continuous Quality Management).

Need of Total Quality Management

The management of all the actions and duties required to uphold the intended standard of excellence within an organisation falls under the purview of TQM. Creating and implementing quality assurance and planning, as well as quality control and improvement programmes, are all included in this.

Additionally, it is utilised to improve customer service, the supply chain management process, and employee training.

Concept of TQM

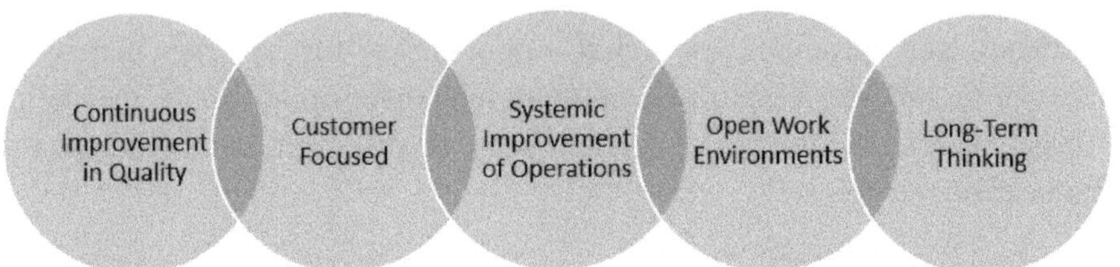

Concept of TQM

The key Concepts of Total Quality Management system are as follows:

1. **Continuous Improvement in Quality**

The TQM system aims to continuously improve the quality of the products and services provided by an organisation. The improvement in quality increases the productivity and thereby improves customer satisfaction and in return helps the organisation establish good control in the market.

2. **Customer Focused**

The TQM system focuses on the customer. The products and services provided should fulfil customer needs and expectations. By focusing on the customer requirements, the organisation can carry out its activities efficiently.

3. **Systemic Improvement of Operations**

The TQM system involves various procedures and processes that are systematic and should comply with the standards.

There should be proper inspection of these processes at regular time intervals and must also be improved and updated duly to meet the required quality levels in the products and services.

4. **Open Work Environments**

For continuous quality improvement, a proper and open work environment for innovation is required where suggestions for improvement are taken and provides an equal opportunity for all the managers, supervisors and the employees to challenge their opinions. It also helps to break barriers amongst the employees of different departments and organisational levels.

5. **Long-Term Thinking**

TQM involves long-term thinking to improve the quality to build the future by understanding the consequences of the current activities. This requires time and discussions based on current problems. Long-Term thinking works best in organisations where the managers share the consequences of their decisions equally.

Principles of TQM

TQM is viewed as a process that prioritises continually improving quality and management while keeping customers in mind. It makes an attempt to ensure that all concerned employees are working toward the same goals of improving the production processes and elevating the calibre of the given goods or services. There are several guiding concepts that characterise TQM.

These are as follows:

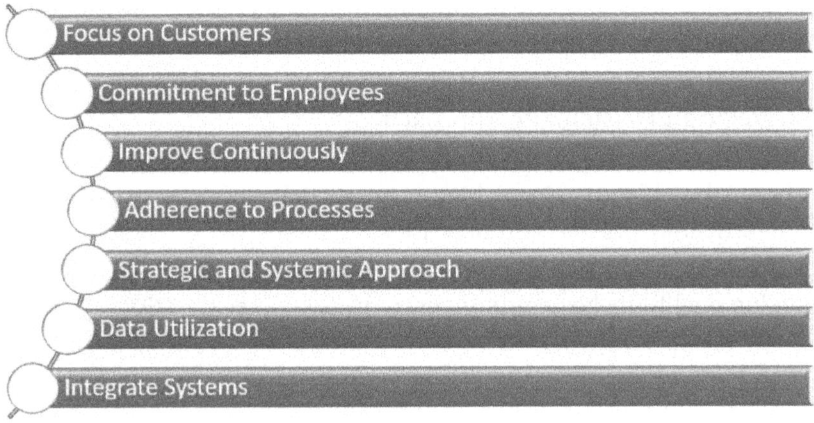

1. **Focus on Customers**

Under TQM, customers decide whether your products are of a high calibre. Customer input is highly valued since it helps a company better understand the requirements and standards for the production process.

2. **Commitment by Employees**

The success of TQM depends on employee support for the policies and system. This entails establishing the goals, expectations, specifications, and restrictions in explicit terms among leaders and across departments.

3. **Improve Continuously**

As a corporation obtains more knowledge about its customers, operations, and competitors, it should gradually alter and strive for small, incremental gains.

This concept of ongoing development allows for greater flexibility in terms of different products, markets, customers, or geographical areas and helps a company adapt to altering consumer expectations.

4. **Adherence to Processes**

TQM's methodical approach commonly uses process flowcharts, TQM diagrams, visual action plans, and documented processes.

5. **Strategic and Systematic Approach**

The goals, objectives, and long-term strategy of a corporation should exactly reflect its policies and practises.

A business must make the appropriate financial investments and commit to making quality its key component in order to execute TQM.

6. **Data Utilization**

The systematic technique of TQM can only be successful if input and feedback are given to evaluate how the process flow is going. Management must continually rely on metrics such as production, turnover, efficiency, and employee data to compare expected and actual results.

7. **Integrate Systems**

Plans for TQM state that systems should talk to one another, share crucial data among departments, and make educated judgments. By linking data sources and exchanging information across systems, TQM attempts to enable everyone to be aware of the same information at the same time.

8. **Communication**

The coordination of processes and ensuring that a full production line operates smoothly involve people, despite how simple it may be to transfer data between departments.

Advantages of TQM

The following are the advantages of TQM:

1. It maintains the quality of the products and services.
2. It strengthens the competitive position.

3. It provides adaptability to changing or emerging market conditions other government regulations.
4. It increases the productivity and profitability.
5. It eliminates defects and waste.
6. It reduces costs and provides better cost management.
7. It improves customer focus and satisfaction.
8. It develops improved and innovative processes.
9. It increases customer loyalty and retention.

Disadvantages of TQM

TQM has the following disadvantages:

1. It demands initial introduction costs, training workers and disrupts the current production while being implemented.
2. The workers of an organisation may be resistant to change and may feel less secure in jobs.
3. It is a long-term process, thus shows results and benefits only after several years.

QUALITY BY DESIGN (QbD)

Introduction

Dr. Joseph M. Juran is the man behind the Quality by Design idea. He held the opinion that a product's quality should be built in from the start and that most quality issues are a result of poor product design. A high-quality drug product is one that is free of contaminants and provides the patient with the appropriate therapeutic benefit, according to Woodcock, a different specialist.

Principles of QbD are implemented in development, manufacturing and regulation of drug products as per USFDA guidelines. According to the FDA, the increased testing does not improve the quality whereas quality should be built into the product. By merging statistical, analytical, and risk-management methodologies into the planning, development, and production of pharmaceutical goods, the QbD approach attempts to ensure the quality of medications.

Objectives of QbD

QbD is a systematic approach that focuses on improving the quality of products based on their design. It mainly emphasises on the design of the product that eventually produces high-quality products and services. It also emphasises on the control of products and processes based on quality risk management.

The main goal of QbD is that the sources of variableness in the processes are identified, studied and managed in an appropriate manner.

The goals of QbD are as follows:

1. To produce high-quality products that meet the standard quality specifications based on clinical performance.
2. To augment the process ability and reduce product variableness and defects by improvising the design, quality, understanding and control of product and processes.
3. To intensify product development and manufacturing competence.
4. To improve post-approval change management and root cause analysis.

QbD blends contemporary process-analytical chemistry techniques with knowledge-management systems to improve the recognition and comprehension of crucial material properties and manufacturing process parameters.

This helps in the production of high-quality products that are accepted widely in the market and meet the required quality and safety specifications. This makes it possible to incorporate quality into the manufacturing process and serves as the foundation for ongoing process and product improvement.

Elements of QbD

To deliver a drug product with such CQAs to the patient, the pharmaceutical QbD approach entails the identification of characteristics that are crucial to quality from the patient's perspective, conversion of those characteristics into drug product critical quality attributes (CQAs), and establishment of a relationship between formulation irregularities and CQAs.

The components of QbD are as follows:

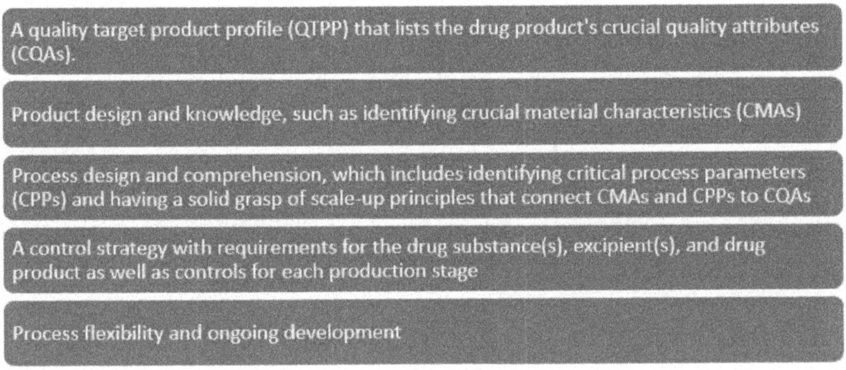

A quality target product profile (QTPP) that lists the drug product's crucial quality attributes (CQAs).

Product design and knowledge, such as identifying crucial material characteristics (CMAs)

Process design and comprehension, which includes identifying critical process parameters (CPPs) and having a solid grasp of scale-up principles that connect CMAs and CPPs to CQAs

A control strategy with requirements for the drug substance(s), excipient(s), and drug product as well as controls for each production stage

Process flexibility and ongoing development

Identifying the Drug Product's Critical Quality Attributes in the Quality Target Product Profile

The QTPP is a projected summary of the quality attributes of a drug product that should be attained in order to assure the desired quality as well as the account safety and effectiveness of the medication product. The design of the product is built upon QTPP. The following should be taken into account for the QTPP's inclusion:

- The intended use, the administration route, the dose form, and the delivery mechanism (s)
- Strength of dose(s)
- System for closing containers

Product Design and Understanding

Products can be designed in a variety of ways because product design is adaptable. Important elements of product design and comprehension include the following:

1. Characterization of the drug substance(s) on a physical, chemical, and biological level.
2. Identification and selection of the type and grade of excipients, as well as knowledge of intrinsic excipient variability.
3. Drug-excipient interactions, formulation improvement, and identification of CMAs for both the excipients and the drug material.

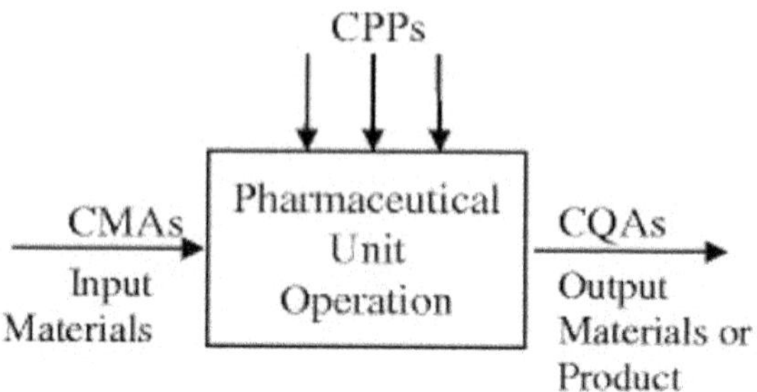

$$CQAs = f\,(CPP_1,\ CPP_2\ ,\ CPP_3\ \ldots CMA_1,\ CMA_2,\ CMA_3\ldots)$$

Control Strategy

- Level 1 uses automatic engineering control to continuously check the quality of the output materials. This is the level of control that is most flexible.
- To ensure that CQAs consistently meet the set acceptance requirements, process parameters are automatically updated, and input material properties are tracked.
- Level 1 control offers a higher level of quality assurance than conventional end-product testing and can enable real-time release testing.
- Level 2 comprises of pharmaceutical control with scaled-back end-product testing, adjustable material attributes, and design-space-conforming process parameters. Finding the sources of variability that have an impact on product quality is made simpler by QbD by encouraging an understanding of the process and the product.
- Level 3 is the level of control traditionally used in the pharmaceutical industry. The rigorous end-product testing, closely controlled material properties, and process parameters used in this control technique.

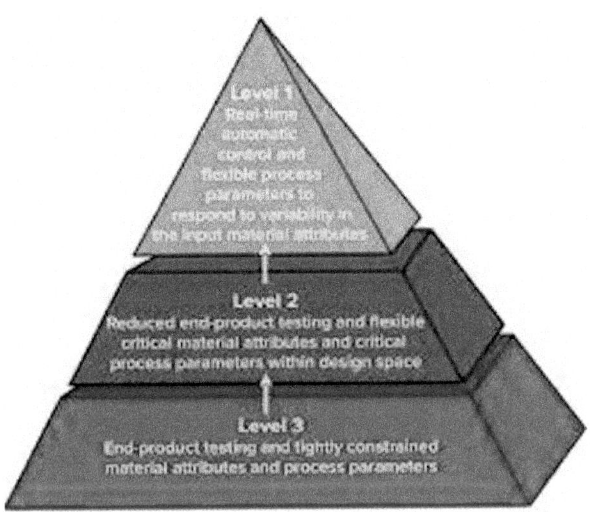

Process Capability and Continual Improvement

The implementation of corrective and preventive measures must be taken when special variances are observed, and this can be done by continuously monitoring the process data for Cpk and other statistical process control measures.

SIX SIGMA CONCEPT

Introduction

Six Sigma Concept is a measurement standard introduced by Carl Frederick Gauss (1777-1855). He gave the concept of normal curve. This concept is being used as a measurement standard since the 1920's where a process requires correction. Later. Many measurement standards were introduced but the term **Six Sigma** was coined by Bill Smith.

The phrase "Six Sigma" refers to a collection of quality-control methods that companies can use to get rid of flaws and enhance procedures in an effort to increase profitability.

The term Six Sigma represents standard deviation that indicates the degree of deviation in the set of measurements or a process or a product. It is a statistical approach used for the measurement of a process or a product in terms of six sigma level as mentioned in Table 1.

Sigma Levels	Defects per Million	Yields
6	3.4	99.99966%
5	230	99.977%
4	6,210	99.38%
3	66,800	93.32%
2	308,000	69.15%
1	690,000	30.85%

Table 1 : Six Sigma Level

Objectives of Six Sigma Concept

The following are the objectives of the Six Sigma Concept:

1. It enhances the level of customer satisfaction.
2. It shortens the time it takes to get a product to market. It reduces defects.
3. It controls variation and improves predictability.
4. Costs are decreased without any unintended repercussions.
5. It enhances measuring and administration of end-to-end proofs.
6. It offers potential to refine current approaches to supply chain improvement.
7. It uses statistical methods to tackle problems in a project-oriented framework.
8. It compares different processes according to the sigma levels. The aim of quality improvement system is to reduce the errors and to maintain them at a low value. Meaning of six sigma is DPMO (Defects per Million Opportunities).

Methodologies

Methodologies of Six Sigma include the key processes, such as **DMAIC** and **DMADV**. The Six Sigma DMAIC process (Define, Measure, Analyze, Improve, and Control) is an improvement system used for the current processes found below specification and looking for incremental improvement. While the Six Sigma DMADV process (Define, Measure, Analyze, Design, and Verify) is also an improvement process used for developing new process or products at Six Sigma quality levels.

The above-mentioned methodologies DMAIC and DMADV are explained in detail below.

1. **DMAIC (Define, Measure, Analyze, Improve, and Control)**

It is a quality strategy that is data-driven and utilized to enhance procedures. The Six Sigma Quality Initiative of the company includes it in full. DMAIC stands for Define, Measure, Analyze, Improve, and Control. These five interconnected steps. In the DMAIC cycle, each step ensures the best possible results.

Following are the process steps of DMAIC:

- **Define:** The client, their Critical to Quality (CTQ) issues, and the business process concerned are defined using the following techniques:

a) Defining customers, their needs, and their expectations in terms of goods and services.
b) Defining the beginning and finish of the project, or its borders.
c) Defining the process to be improved by mapping the process flow.

- **Measure:** The following metrics are used to assess how well the business process involved is performing:

a) Developing a data collection plan for the process.
b) Obtaining information from various sources to identify the different kinds of problems and metrics.
c) Comparing to consumer surveys to identify gaps.

- **Analyze:** To identify the primary causes of errors and areas for development, it analyses the gathered data and process map in the following ways:

a) Identifying the gaps between current performance and the performance to be achieved.
b) Prioritizing opportunities for the improvement.
c) Identifying the sources of variation.

- **Improve:** It prevents and fixes problems of targeting by designing creative solutions in the following ways:

a) Creating innovative solutions with the help of technology and discipline.

b) Creating and planning an implementation strategy.

- **Control:** In the following ways, it regulates improvements to maintain the novelty of the process:

a) Preventing the process from reverting back to the old way.

b) Developing, documenting and implementing the current monitoring process.

c) Institutionalizing the improvement by modifying the systems and structures (staffing, training, incentives).

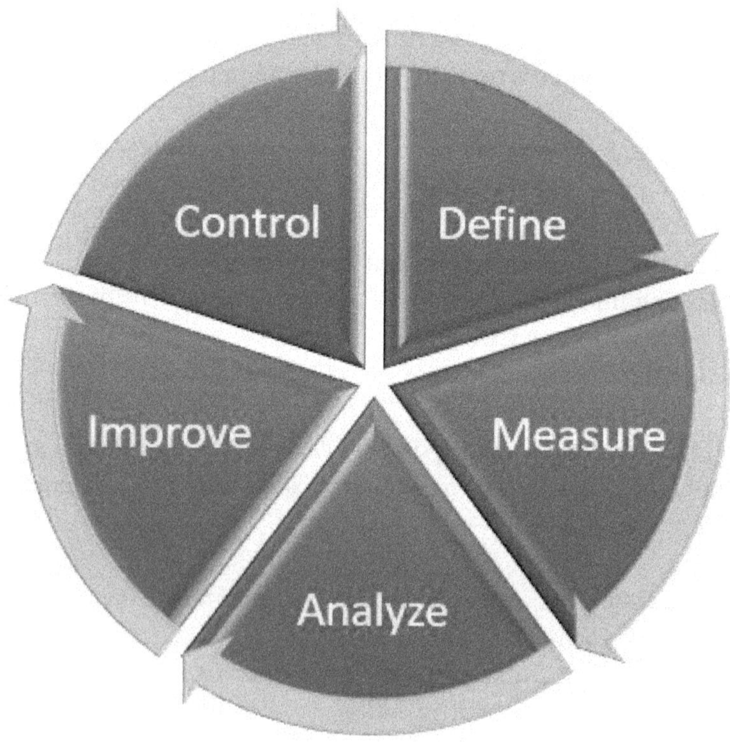

DMAIC

2. **DMADV(Define, Measure, Analyze, Design, and Verify)**

It is an abbreviated form of Define, Measure, Analyze, Design, and Verify. It is a system of improvement used for developing new processes or products at Six Sigma quality levels.

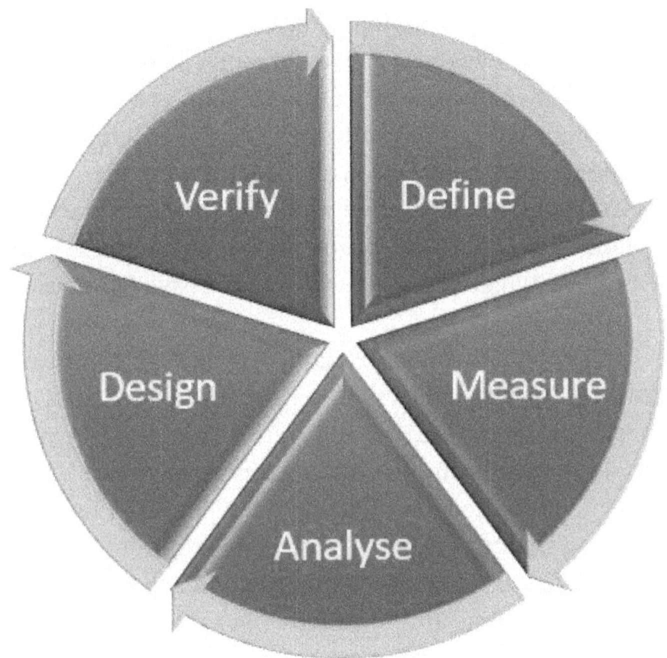

DMADV

Similarities between DMAIC and DMADV

DMAIC and DMADV are both:

1) Methods of Six Sigma are employed to decrease flaws with a probability of 34 or less per million opportunities.

2) Data-intensive problem-solving techniques.

3) Carried out by Green Belts. Master Black Belts and Black Belts.

4) Helps to achieve the bottom-line financial and/or commercial goals.

5) Used to implement the support of a champion and process owner.

Applications in Pharmaceutical Industry

The pharmaceutical companies have adopted the concept of six sigma in the past few years for reducing cycle time and cost. To launch a six sigma within pharmaceutical industry, the following key strategies are suggested:

1. Six Sigma is used to promote the adoption of necessary integration initiatives with a commitment from top-down leadership, changing the conventional methods of conducting clinical trials.
2. Six Sigma is used to integrate the technology and to improve the workflow in meeting challenges as well as to start new ventures which cannot be initiated using conventional isolated implementation of technology or home-grown process improvement methods.
3. Six Sigma gives trustworthy, tried-and-true research methods for evaluating quantitatively clinical development and process-improving initiatives, which are integrated in line with impressive financial success.

Application of Six Sigma can be explained by giving the example of supplier and material approval process in a company's packaging division. The entire process of identification and certification of a supplier of packaging materials is highly complex, and thus normally takes 12 months. This process can be simplified by forming a Six Sigma team of 4 pilot products, determining the critical paths, and analyzing and identifying the problems involved in the process. Six Sigma methodology also helped the team to streamline the process and to reduce the cycle time from 12 to 5 months, thus making the process less time-consuming.

OUT OF SPECIFICATIONS (OOS)

Introduction

The term Out of Specifications (OOS) is employed for testing results that fall outside the parameters listed in compendia, drug master files, or drug applications for finished products or in-process samples. The 00S may be brought about by mistakes made during the testing process, variations in the production process, or poor analytical tools. Investigating the causes of OOS should be done via a root cause analysis.

OOS causes can be divided into **assignable** and **non-assignable** categories. It is deemed to be **outside of specifications** if the limitations go outside of the range given. The analyst should let the OC management know if OOS has happened. The senior management should then request from QA to send an OOS form to the analyst. The OOS investigation involves two phases:

- **Phase I or Laboratory Investigation**

Laboratory investigation is mainly performed to identify the reasons due to which OOS occur. Defects in the production process or the measuring method could be among the causes.

Regardless of the rejection of batches, the results obtained from OOS should investigate for their trend.

The investigation should be carried out on the batches that produced OOS, as well as on other batches and related items.

The OOS inquiry needs to be carried out completely, promptly, objectively, well recorded, and scientifically.

Before discarding the test and standard preparations, the phase I investigations should be thoroughly performed.

In phase I investigation, it is necessary to analyze the root cause and to recognize the error that may have resulted due to:

1) Standard and sample solution dilution error,
2) Errors in the analyzing process,
3) Equipment failure, and
4) Calculation error.

1. **Phase 1a Investigation**

In this phase of investigation mistakes such as miscalculations or power outages, as well as testing faults such spills or erroneous equipment parameter setup, are recognized. These problems are anticipated to persist even if a laboratory study 1b or 2 was negative.

2. **Phase 1b Investigation**

It is the starting phase of investigation, which is performed by the analyst and supervisor using the laboratory investigation checklist including the related areas of investigation.

In the guidance details of checks, the following checklist documented are considered:

1) Proper test methods were used, e.g., Version number.
2) Correctly chosen/tested sample(s) (whether or not the check labels were taken from correct place).

3) Maintenance of chain of custody, proper container, and sample integrity (was there an unusual event or problem).

Only data/equipment analysis review should be undertaken as the first step of the investigation by the analyst and supervisor.

After performing the initial review, re-measurement is performed to support the investigation testing this is done only alters the documentation of hypothesis plan.

Investigative testing or a hypothesis can support or refute a potential root cause. Additional testing for the sample, filtration, sonication/ extraction, equipment failure, etc. is included in this testing. It is possible to investigate more than one hypothesis during the study.

A different preparation from the original sample cannot be used in the initial hypothesis testing, but the original functioning stock solutions can.

A test can be cancelled if a clear root cause has been determined, such as:

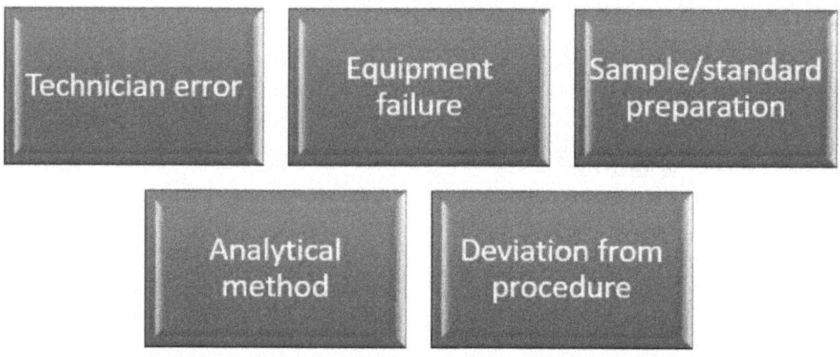

Phase II Investigation

The phase I investigation should be performed if no possible outcome is obtained from phase I investigation. This phase of investigation is performed to identify the errors that occurred in manufacturing processes, sampling procedures, along with other additional laboratory testing.

When phase I investigation fails to identify a detectable laboratory error, phase II investigation is carried out.

These investigations should always be conducted in conjunction with a manufacturing investigation to ascertain whether there was a potential manufacturing root cause.

They are based on written and approved instructions against hypotheses. Details on resampling, retesting, averaging, and written description are also included in the written instructions.

Before beginning an investigative test, the entire testing process should be documented out in detail and authorized by QA or a QA equivalent.

- **Phase III Investigation**

Once the batch is rejected another batch is investigated to determine whether or not the other batches or products are affected.

The factors related to validation methods and possible causes into fluctuations in the results are also investigated. The recommendations further state that if a batch is rejected, additional testing should be carried out to identify the root cause of failure and allow for the implementation of corrective measures. Furthermore, the rejection decision cannot be changed because of additional testing.

To ascertain the effect of OOS results on other batches, ongoing stability studies, verified processes, and testing procedures, quality control (QC) and quality assurance (QA) approaches are used. The conclusion reached by QC and DA, as well as the necessary corrective and preventive measures, are documented.

Once a comprehensive examination has revealed that the OS results are not indicative of the quality of the batch, a final decision about the release of a batch (despite an initial 0OS result that was not invalidated) should be made.

Concluding the Investigation

Once OOS has been verified through examination, batch failure investigation may follow. Other batches and other products may be the subject of these investigations. The batches that OOS has certified will be thoroughly documented and destroyed.

In case the results are not confirmed by 0OS, the quality assurance department will take decision to release the batch.

Whole investigation can be concluded in the following points:

1) The analytical method, sampling procedure, and dilutions were discovered to be reliable and validated during phase I of the laboratory testing study.

2) The inquiry then moves on to phase II, where all manufacturing processes were found to be reliable and additional testing to be reliable.

3) Subsequent QA reveals that the initial OOS did not accurately represent the batch's quality.

CHANGE CONTROL

Introduction

Change Control is a CGMP concept that successfully avoids unintended consequences After regulatory filings and earlier regulatory documentation, some manufacturing adjustments (such as those that modify the requirements, a crucial product attribute, or bioavailability) may be made.

The life cycle of a pharmaceutical product must include change control. A change occurs when a manufacturing facility, facilities, process, material, product, procedure, or piece of equipment (including software) is added, removed, or modified and has an impact on the quality or regulatory requirements.

Change control procedures ensure that adjustments are made in a planned and well-coordinated way. The drug product, intermediate, or API production and control modifications are all evaluated by the change control program. It is the most important component of pharmaceutical business quality management.

By monitoring, evaluating, and approving the modifications, a change control system balances and verifies the quality system. Insufficient change control methods lead to regulatory non-compliance.

Change management seeks to stop unforeseen consequences from occurring when a system or product is changed.

Benefits of Change Control System

The following are the benefits of the Change Control System:

1. Improved Productivity

According to research, the typical employee only works three productive hours every day. One of the major reasons for this behaviour is unclear deliverables or the poorly managed execution process. Change control frequently resolves this problem by lessening employee uncertainty around project deliverables, hence enhancing general staff productivity.

2. Collaborative Teamwork

By compiling all the project information in one place, the change control process speeds the implementation. Additionally, it aids in fostering effective team communication, facilitating smooth collaboration across cross-functional teams on change initiatives.

3. Effective Change Communication

Transparency in change management communication is essential to getting your team on board with impending changes and helping everyone in the organisation embrace them. Utilizing effective change communication will enable you to address diverse resistance factors and overcome internal resistance.

4. Decreased Cost of Change

The chance of a change effort failing is successfully reduced and minimised through the change control process. The streamlined strategy optimises resources and lowers project expenses.

5. It helps in documenting and tracking the details of change.

6. It provides structured and systematic approach for change management with proper change evaluation.

7. It demonstrates compliance to regulatory agencies

Change Control Procedure

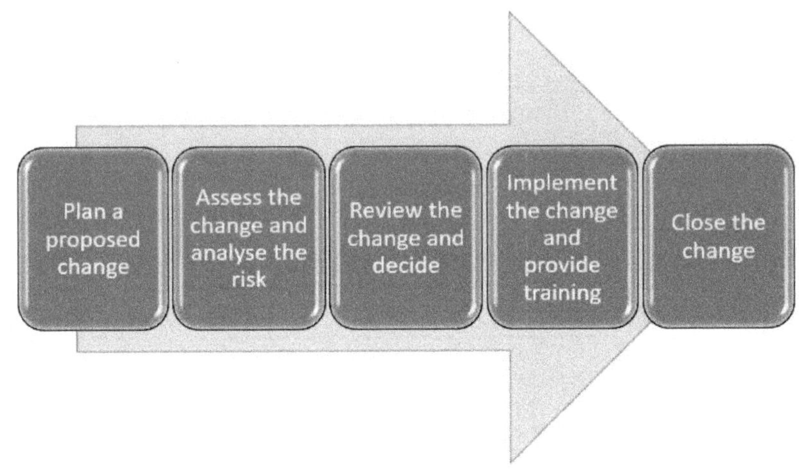

Change Control Steps

ISO 9000 SERIES FOR QUALITY SYSTEMS AND STANDARDS

Introduction

International quality assurance and management standards are outlined in ISO 9000. The International Organization for Standardization ISO created and released the ISO 9000 set of standards. For manufacturing and service businesses, it defines, creates, and maintains an efficient quality assurance QA system.

It has been formulated to help the companies in efficiently documenting the quality system elements to be incorporated so that an effective quality system can be maintained.

A corporation may satisfy customers, adhere to regulations, and continually develop with the aid of ISO 9000. It is not a complete assurance of quality, merely the initial phase or the foundational level of a quality system.

The ISO 9000 standard is well-known worldwide. It seeks to implement a QMS into an organization to boost efficiency, cut wasteful expenditure, and guarantee the quality of products and procedures.

As a manual for high-quality goods, services, and management, it benefits numerous diverse industries and organizations.

ISO 9000 series of Standards

The ISO 9000 family contains these standards:

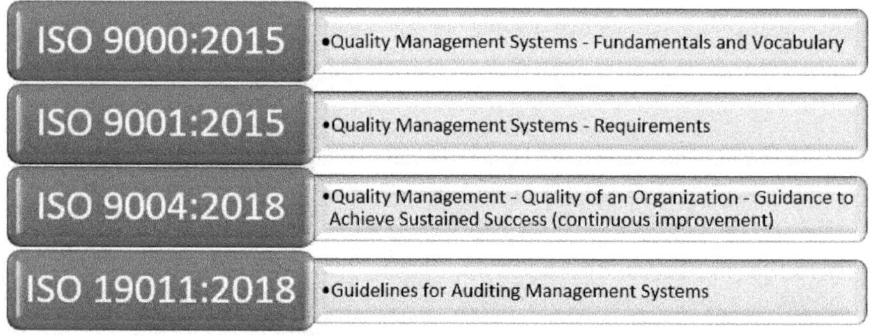

Fig 1.15

Principles of ISO 9000 Family

The seven quality management principles included in ISO 9000 Family are:

Customer Focus
Relationship Management
Engagement of People
Quality Management Principles
Evidence-based Decision Making
Leadership and Continuous Improvement
Process Approach

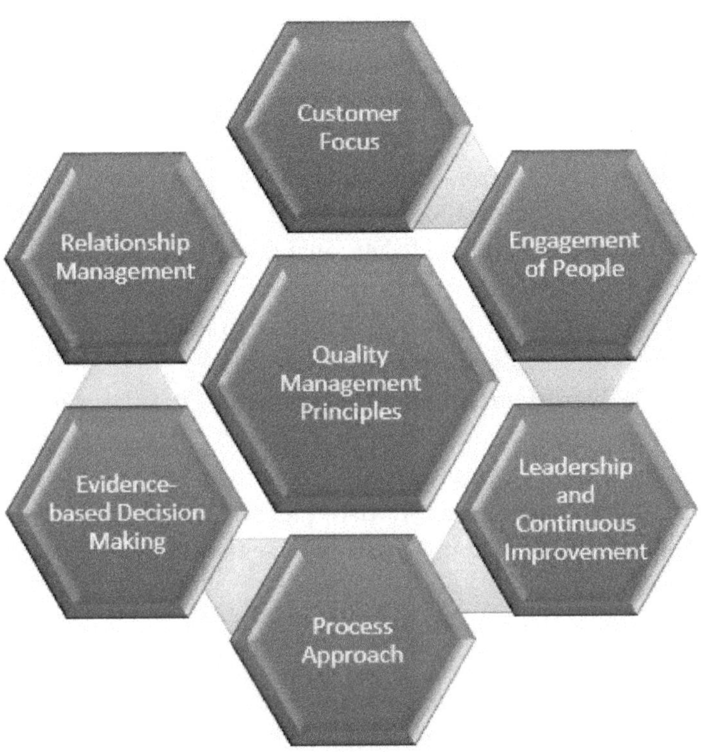

Principles of ISO 9000 Family

1. **Customer Focus:** Businesses must be conscious of what customers want and make an extra effort to satisfy them. Businesses should gauge how satisfied customers are with their goods or services. Surveys are one method to accomplish this, and another is to keep an eye on consumer complaints.
2. **Leadership:** The future of the company should be envisioned by organisational leaders, who should also provide employees with the resources they need to realise that vision. Leaders should build rapport with their team members and value their efforts.

3. **Process Approach:** Resources should be managed by organisations as a process. They ought to evaluate the company's capabilities using process analysis tools, look for ways to connect operations to make processes simpler, and assess the efficiency of processes.
4. **Continuous Improvement:** Businesses should have a perpetual improvement strategy, empower employees to make changes, track changes systematically, and recognise them.
5. **Engagement:** Employees at every level should be involved.
6. **Evidence-based Decision-Making:** Decisions made by organisations should be supported by solid data analysis, practical experience, and qualitative evidence. This entails the use of methods like multi-voting, which aids a group in reducing a list of possibilities, and decision matrices to rank and assess options.
7. **Relationship Management:** The development of profitable partnerships with partner organisations, such as suppliers, service providers, and contractors, should be a top priority for businesses. They must pool resources, collaborate on R&D initiatives, and recognise success in order to implement effective supply chain management.

Significance of ISO 9000 Family

- It offers guidelines for how a company's product or service will satisfy stakeholder and consumer expectations while still adhering to regulatory obligations.
- It assists a company in creating, maintaining, and constantly enhancing its QMS with the aim of delivering the highest possible service or product quality.
- Businesses who adhere to the rules are expected to see a decrease in production costs as a result of the standards and controls put in place, which limit the likelihood of expensive and time-consuming errors. Organizations may employ workers, resources, and time more effectively by concentrating on the process. Because compliance improves an organization's reputation, adhering to the rules can provide firms a competitive edge.

Working

A corporation may use ISO 9000's collection of best practices to set up, maintain, and enhance its quality management system. Organizations have the freedom to apply the quality management system in their own efficient method because ISO 9000 is not a fixed set of guidelines. This freedom enables various organizations and large and small businesses to use the ISO 9000 standard.

An ISO 9001 certification may increase a company's reputation by demonstrating to clients that the company's goods and services are up to par. Additionally, there are specific circumstances in which companies in some industries are compelled by law to have an ISO 9001 certification.

To obtain ISO 9001 certification, a company must exhibit the qualities listed below:

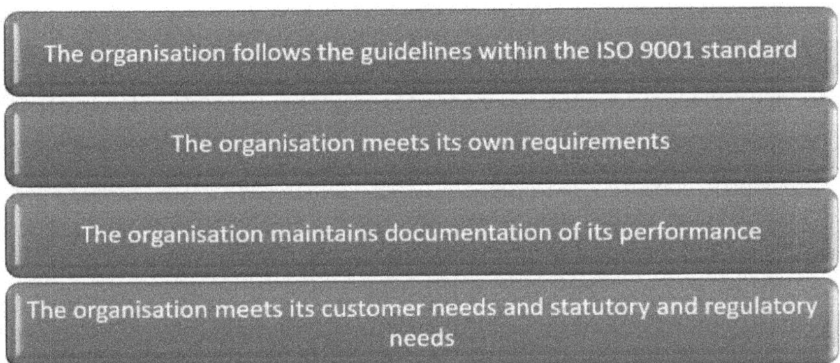

ISO 14000

Introduction

The ISO 14000 family of standards provides practical tools for different companies and organizations who desire to manage their environmental responsibilities. ISO 14000 and its supporting standards focus on environmental systems to achieve this.

The additional ISO 14000 standards are centered on environmental concerns including climate change, communications, labeling, life cycle analysis, and audits.

ISO 14000 is applicable for the following:

- Any organization (single-site to large MNCs, high risk to low-risk companies).

- The manufacturing industries (equipment manufacturers and suppliers), process industries, and service industries.
- All industries of local government, public and private sectors.

The basic features of ISO 14000 are:

- Minimum harmful effects on the environment.
- Continuous improvement to achieve the desired performances.

Principles

The principle of ISO 14000 is explained by **PDCA Model**.

- **Plan:** Designing of aim, objective, and processes to achieve the desired result.
- **Do:** The designed process should be performed step by step. The changes are noted and data is stored to analyse the results.
- **Check:** The evaluation of the data and results recorded in the previous steps.
- **Act:** The evaluation of the data and results helps to improve the process. In this step, the problems of the result are rectified for continuous improvement and for this purpose, Do and Check steps may be repeated several times for a better outcome. The causes of the difference in the results are identified and improved. This step is often named 'Adjust'.

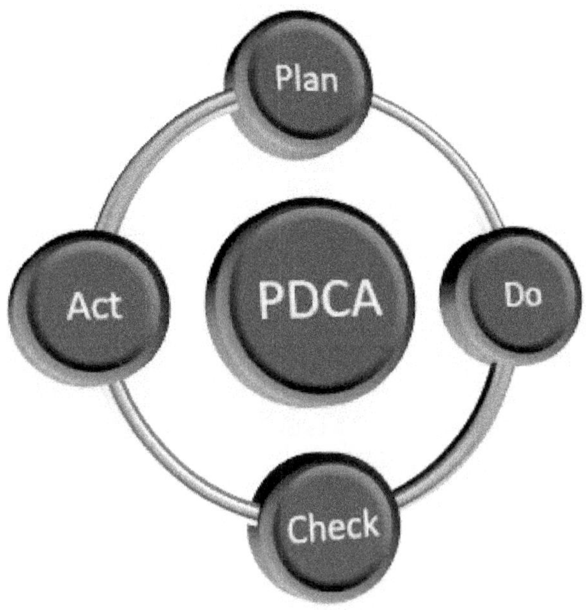

ISO 14000 Series

ISO 14000 includes the following standards. The most important standard is ISO 14001 that gives guidelines for implementation of Environmental Management System (EMS).

ISO 14004 is another significant standard which gives additional information and specialized standards for implementation of EMS.

The key standards included in ISO 14000 are as follows:

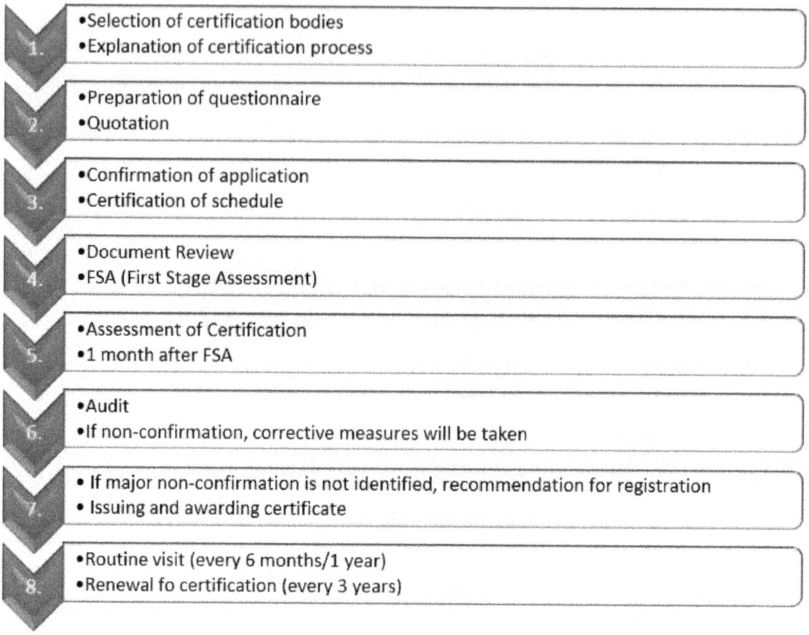

1.
- Selection of certification bodies
- Explanation of certification process

2.
- Preparation of questionnaire
- Quotation

3.
- Confirmation of application
- Certification of schedule

4.
- Document Review
- FSA (First Stage Assessment)

5.
- Assessment of Certification
- 1 month after FSA

6.
- Audit
- If non-confirmation, corrective measures will be taken

7.
- If major non-confirmation is not identified, recommendation for registration
- Issuing and awarding certificate

8.
- Routine visit (every 6 months/1 year)
- Renewal fo certification (every 3 years)

Process of ISO 14001 Certification

Benefits of ISO 14000 Certification

This certification helps organizations to maintain their conformation to the environmental regulations in the following ways:

- Better marketability.
- Better utilization of resources.
- Environmental responsibilities.
- Better quality of finished goods and products.
- Customers' satisfaction.
- Enhancement of the reputation and reliability of the organization.

GOOD LABORATORY PRACTICES (GLP) & NATIONAL ACCREDITATION BOARD FOR TESTING AND CALIBRATION LABORATORIES (NABL)

GOOD LABORATORY PRACTICES (GLP)

Introduction

Good Laboratory Practice (GLP) should be followed in pharmaceutical laboratories. The key factors to take into account under GLP are listed below:

- To accommodate the performance of all quality control tests and analyses, the laboratory should be situated, designed, customised, and maintained.
- • In order to safeguard the fragile instruments, it should be situated in a convenient location to serve the manufacturing department but apart from it to prevent vibration, dust, and internal and external traffic.
- There should be separate wings for analytical, instruments, microbiology, sterility, etc., which should be connected with the internal door.
- • There should be a fumigation chamber, an efficient airlock, and equipment for air conditioning. The laboratory should be adequately sized and equipped with utilities, storage for water and solvents, extraction dust collection, etc.
- The laboratory furniture should provide adaptability. The table top should be covered with material that is resistant to acids, alkali, solvents, etc.

Equipment

- Standard operating procedures for every instrument must be outlined in writing. The instrument needs to be kept tidy at all times and put in an appropriate spot in a separate, temperature-controlled room. Additionally, it needs to be handled very carefully. Additionally, the surroundings needed to be cleansed.
- Records of calibration, maintenance, and servicing must be preserved and updated on a regular basis.
- Before use, the glassware must be calibrated with a certified one. Glassware that is intended to be used for measuring purposes, in particular, has to be calibrated before use.
- All relevant operating, handling, and care instructions should be visible next to the equipment. There should be enough light.

.

Chemicals and Reagents

- Chemicals and reagents should be stored in a way that involves their usage, and all of their containers need to be clearly labelled.
- Chemical transfers must be handled with extreme caution.
- A prepared solution and all analytical reagents need to be labelled.
- Molar Solution records entered in the register created for the purpose.

Organization and Personnel

- Every person working in the lab and conducting tests must have the necessary educational requirements and have the necessary training and experience to carry out their assigned duties.
- To execute the research correctly and in line with procedures, there must be an adequate number of staff. To prevent contaminating the test and control objects in the test systems, the workers must take the necessary safeguards.
- The staff should be given attire that is appropriate for their needs and made from natural materials to prevent contamination from microorganisms and chemicals.
- To make sure that they won't be a source of contamination and to assess their health, the staff should undergo a thorough medical check.
- The laboratory should have a clearly defined organ gram, and responsibilities and obligations at all levels should be clearly stated and recorded.

Documentation

- The paperwork is essential to a successful laboratory. Practice documentation is the established technique for storing data for later use.
- Protocols, logbooks for equipment use, maintenance, and calibration, and well-established SOPs are the essential documentation that must be provided.

Protocols and Conduct of a Laboratory Test

- To conduct the test, each laboratory should create a well-defined protocol that specifically states.

Quality Control

- There needs to be a clear process in place that addresses every component of the sample, including the consignment's reception, the sampling methods to be used, sample handling and storage, recording, and analysis reporting.
- Each received sample needs to have a unique number, which should be written on the sample's label and kept in the correct storage environment.
- A clear sample procedure must be in place, and it must expressly and precisely describe the sampling procedure. What number of samples can be blended together, if it is allowed, etc.

Records and Reports

- Every laboratory should keep track of all the tests run, and any graphs related to IR, HPLC, etc. should be kept alongside the raw data. Access to records should be limited to those who are permitted, and they should ideally be kept under lock and key for rapid reference.

Safety

- The necessary equipment for fire extinguishing in the event of an accident, as well as proper facilities and accessories, should be available to ensure the safety of the workers involved in drug testing.

NATIONAL ACCREDITATION BOARD FOR TESTING AND CALIBRATION LABORATORIES (NABL)

The Department of Science & Technology, Government of India, oversees the National Accreditation Board for Testing and Calibration Laboratories (NABL), an independent organisation whose goal is to accredit the testing and calibration of clinical laboratories throughout the nation.

A constituent board of the Quality Council of India is the NABL. Its objective is to offer the government, business associations, and industry a system of accreditation for conformity assessment bodies that involves independent evaluation of the technical proficiency of testing by organisations like calibration and medical labs, proficiency testing companies, and producers of reference materials.

Additionally, NABL has connections to both the International Laboratory Accreditation Cooperation and the Asia Pacific Laboratory

Accreditation Cooperation. The requirements of the Mutual Recognition Arrangements (MRAs), of which NABL is a member, are also taken into account by the NABL accreditation system.

All significant branches of science and engineering, including Biological, Chemical, Electrical, Electronics, Mechanical, and Fluid-Flow, are accredited by NABL. Testing facilities include non-destructive, photometry, radiological, thermal, and forensics, while calibration facilities include electro-technical, mechanical, and radiological. It also provides accreditation for medical testing laboratories. It provides accreditation for proficiency testing providers and reference material producers.

Conclusion

This report discusses about the 'Recent Advancements in the Quality Management Systems'. The project is centred on the Quality Management System (QMS) and latest developments in QM approaches, which deal with adequate documentation of policies, processes, procedures, and controls to produce high-quality goods and services that satisfy customers' expectations and exceed industry standards. It also discusses the requirement for certifications like ISO 9000 and ISO 14000 as well as the numerous certifications necessary for a standard QM System to function basically. Additionally, the project contains several QMS components, such as TQM, QbD, Six Sigma Concept, OOS, and Change Control. The project provides information about NABL, whose mission is to accredit clinical laboratories nationwide for testing and calibration. It talks about Good Laboratory Practises which are necessary for laboratories to operate correctly and consistently.

References

Books

- Dr. Ilango K.B., Dr. Vikesh Kumar Shukla, Dr. Sameer H. Lakade: Industrial Pharmacy-II: Chapter-7: Quality Management Systems: Thakur Publications Pvt. Ltd.: Lucknow
- Dr. K.P. Sampath Kumar, Dr. Debjit Bhowmik, Rishab Bhanot, Shambaditya Goswami: Industrial Pharmacy-II: First Edition: Chapter-4: Quality Management Systems: Nirali Publications

Submitted Works

- JCB Academy on 2019-02-15

- University of Johannesburg on 2019-05-27
- De Montfort University on 2022-09-11
- Institute of Technology Carlow on 2021-12-12
- Colorado Technical University Online on 2015-04-29
- University of Petroleum and Energy Studies on 2019-08-23
- University of Huddersfield on 2022-07-02
- Nelson Mandela Metropolitan University on 2021-10-22
- University of Greenwich on 2020-05-18
- Intercollege on 2022-09-26
- University of Greenwich on 2020-05-18
- Pacific University on 2021-08-27
- Philippine Council for Health Research and Development on 2020-08-02
- London School of Marketing on 2017-07-04
- CSU, Dominguez Hills on 2022-04-07

CHAPTER V

UNIT 5 Indian Regulatory Requirements

At the end of the chapter, student will understand and gain knowledge about :

Indian Regulatory Requirements: Central Drug Standard Control Organization (CDSCO) and State Licensing Authority: Organization, Responsibilities, Certificate of Pharmaceutical Product (COPP), Regulatory requirements and approval procedures for New Drugs.

Indian Regulatory Requirements

Central drug standard control organization (CDSCO) and State licensing authority: organization, responsibilities, certificate of pharmaceutical product (COPP), Regulatory requirements and approval procedures for new drugs.

Introduction

In India, regulatory requirements with respect to drugs, cosmetics and medical devices are governed by the Drugs and Cosmetics Act 1940 and rules 1945. The requirements of GMP and GLP have further enforced Stringent provisions. Other important legislations include the Narcotics and Psychotropic Substances Act and Rules, The Drugs (Prices Control) Order, the Patents Act and the Designs Act. Throughout the current international scenario, educators must be familiar with the regulatory guidelines issued by the WHO, the US FDA, and other similar organizations in order to be prepared to face global challenges. This chapter attempts to familiarize students with current Indian regulatory requirements for drugs, cosmetics, and medical devices.

Central drug standard control organization (CDSCO)

The Drugs and Cosmetics Act of 1940 and the Rules of 1945 entrusted various responsibilities for drug and cosmetic regulation to central and state regulators. It considers uniform implementation of the Act's and Rules' provisions for ensuring the safety, rights, and well-being of patients by regulating drugs and cosmetics. CDSCO is constantly striving to improve transparency, accountability, and consistency in its services in order to ensure the safety, efficacy, and quality of medical products manufactured, imported, and distributed in the country.

CDSCO is responsible under the Drugs and Cosmetics Act for the approval of drugs, the conduct of clinical trials, the establishment of drug standards, the control of the quality of imported drugs in the country, and the coordination of the activities of State Drug Control Organizations by providing expert advice in order to achieve uniformity in the enforcement of the Drugs and Cosmetics Act.

Furthermore, CDSCO, in collaboration with state regulators, is responsible for granting licenses for certain specialized categories of critical drugs, such as blood and blood products, intravenous fluids, vaccines, and sera.

- The Central Drug Standard Control Organization (CDSCO) is the main regulatory body of India for regulation of **Pharmaceutical, Medical devices and Clinical trials.**
- CDSCO is the Central Drug Authority for discharging function assigned to the Central Government under the Drug and Cosmetics Act 1940 and rules 1945.
- Head office of CDSCO is located in New Delhi
- Functioning under the Control of Directorate General of Health Services, Ministry of Health and Family Welfare, Government of India.
- **Vision:**
- To protect and promote health in India.
- **Mission:**
- To safeguard and enhance the public health by assuring to safety, efficacy and quality of drugs, cosmetics and medical devices.

ORGANIZATION OF CDSCO

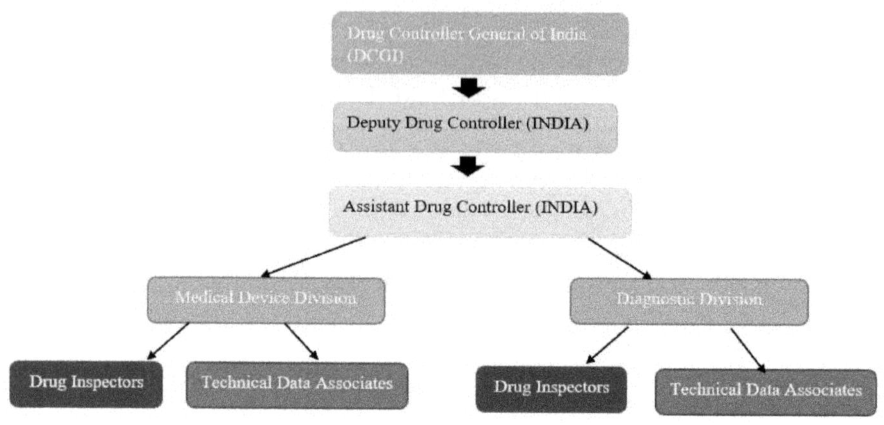

Drug Controller General of India (DCGI)

- He/she is a responsible for approval of **New Drugs, Medical devices and Clinical Trials** to be conducted in India.
- He is appointed by the Central Government under the State Drug Control Organization will be functioning.
- The DCGI is advised by the Drug Technical Advisory Board (DTAB) and the Drug Consultative Committee (DCC).

Responsibilities and Functions of CDSCO

- **Statutory functions:**

1. Forms standards of drugs, cosmetics, diagnostics and devices.
2. Regulatory measures, amendments to Acts and Rules.
3. To regulate market authorization of new drugs.
4. To regulate clinical research in India.
5. To approve licenses to manufacture certain categories of drugs as Central Licence approving Authority i.e., for Blood Banks, Large volume parenteral and Vaccines and Sera.
6. To regulate the standards of imported drugs.
7. Works relating to the DTAB and DCC.
8. Testing of drugs by Central Drugs Labs.

9. Publication of Indian Pharmacopoeia.

- Other Functions:

1. Coordinating the activities of the State Drug Control Organizations to achieve uniform Administration of the Act and policy guidance.
2. Guidance on technical matters.
3. Participation in the WHO GMP certification scheme.
4. Monitoring adverse drug reactions (ADR)
5. Conducting training programmes for regulatory officials and Govt. Analysts.
6. Distribution of quotas of narcotic drugs for use in medicinal formulations.
7. Screening of drug formulations available in Indian market.
8. Evaluation/screening of applications for granting No objection certificates for export of unapproved/banned drugs.

STATE LICENSING AUTHORITY

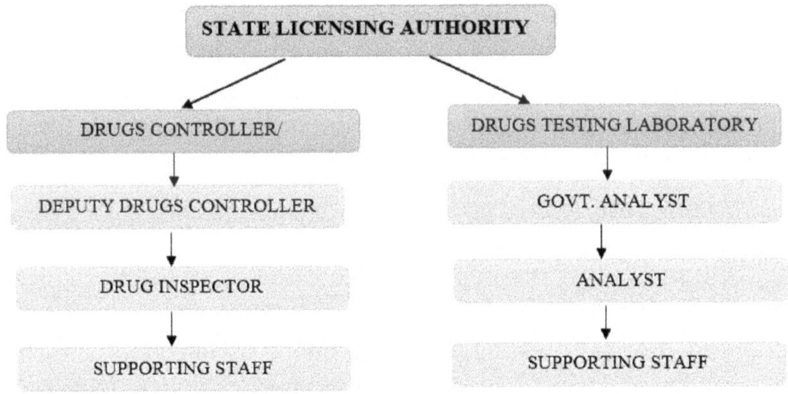

STATE LICENSING AUTHORITY

Responsibilities and functions of SDCO

- Licensing of drug manufacturing and sales establishments.
- Licensing of drug testing laboratories.
- Approval of drug formulations for manufacture.

- Monitoring of quality of Drugs & Cosmetics, manufactured by respective state units and those marketed in the state.
- Investigation and prosecution in respect of contravention of legal provisions.
- Administrative actions.
- Pre and post licensing inspection.
- Recall of sub-standard drugs.

CERTIFICATE OF PHARMACEUTICAL PRODUCT (COPP)

- The COPP certificate is given by the **National Health Authorities** upon demand from the client, the specialists or the producer of item.
- A COP is in the format recommended by the **WHO**.
- It is the importing country who requires the COPP for the pharmaceutical product and a special type of certificate which enables a given pharmaceutical product to be registered and marketed in the exporting country of interest and forms parts of the marketing authorization application.
- This is issued by the Inspectorate and the fabricator of the product having GMP position and also the position of the pharmaceutical, radiopharmaceutical, biological or veterinary product.
- The approved information for different pharmaceutical forms and strengths is varied so it is always issued for a single product.

AIM:

A COPP shows that the imported medication is of the fitting standard of value, security and adequacy to permit it in their market, having experienced thorough testing and assessment to Regulatory Authorities in the trading nation and furthermore exhibits that it follows the right rules and techniques of Good Manufacturing Practice (GMP), expanding the degree of value and without a doubt wellbeing of the item.

SCOPE:

- It is needed when the product is intended for **registration or its renewal** (licensing, authorization or prolongation) by the importing country, with the scope that the product is distributed or commercialized in that country.

- A certificate has been recommended so that it helps the undersized Drug Regulatory authorities (DRA) or also without proper quality assurance facilities in importing countries by WHO and also it can assess the pharmaceutical products quality as per the requirements of importation or registration.

INSPECTION:

The DRA gives a COPP only after conducting an inspection of the manufacturing product.

TYPES OF COPP

1. **WHO 1975 type COPP:**

The WHO 1975 version is a certificate to be issued by exporting country regulatory authority stating:

- The authorized product has to be placed on the market for its use in the country also, the permit number and issue date or
- That the nonauthorized product has placed on the market for its use in the country and also adds the reasons why it is needed;
- As recommended by WHO, the manufacturer of product conforms to GMP requirements.
- Only within the country of origin the products to be sold or distributed or
- To be exported to manufacturing plant where the product is produced and at suitable intervals subject to inspections.

2. WHO 1988 type COPP

The competent authority of the exporting country should have:

- All labelling copies
- Product detailed information in the country of origin

3. WHO 1992 type COPP

This is intended for use by the competent authority of an importing country in two situations:

- When the question arises related to importation and sale license and

- For license renew, extend, review or changes.

FORMAT:

This certificate conforms to the format recommended by WHO

- Certificate No.:
- Importing country (requesting) name:
- Exporting country (certifying) name:

1. Name and its dosage form:

1.1 API(s) and its amount per dose

1.2 Is the product placed for use in the exporting country or not?

1.3 If the product present on the market in the exporting country?

- If the answer is yes, continue with section and omit section 3.
- If the answer is no, omit section 2 and continue with section 3.

1. Number of product license and date of issue:

2.2 Product license holder (name and address):

1. Status of product license holder:

2.3.1. For b and c categories, the name of product and address of its manufacturer must be present:

2.4 If approval appended or not?

2.5 Is the officially approved product information complete and readily available according to the license?

2.6 Applicant for certificate, if different from license holder (name and address):

3. Certificate applicant (name, address and required info);

3.1 Status of applicant:

3.2 For (b) and (c) categories, the name and address of the manufacturer producing the dosage form is:

3.3 If the marketing authorization not required, not requested, under consideration or refused?

3.4 Other additional information

3.5 If the periodic inspection of the manufacturing plant in which the dosage form is produced or not/ not applicable?

If not or not applicable, proceed to question 5;4. Routine inspections periodicity (years):

4.1 Has the manufacture been inspected or not?

4.2 The operations and facilities conform to GMP recommendation or not?

5. The information submitted by the applicant satisfy the certifying authority or not?

Explanation required if not authorized:

1. certifying authority address:
2. Fax:
3. Telephone:
4. Name of authorized person with signature:
5. Stamp or date:

How to obtain COPP?

- To obtain a COPP, a request is made to the exporting country's health authority by the Marketing Authorization Holder (MAH).
- An authorized person issues the COPP and returns it to the MAH. Also, other documents required to obtain a COPP including an application for Export Certificate form, evidence of a GMP certificate (if applicable), Manufacturing License and the last approved SmPC (Summary pf Product Characteristics).

Certificates May Be Issued

- Legally marketable drug in the country.
- Nonauthorized drugs for distribution in the country which are legally exported
- For a foreign manufactured drug. Exportation for personal use
- Awareness is necessary for the drugs that are legal in some countries may be illegal in other countries.

Importation for personal use

- Risky to health, such drugs are prevented from importation.
- Also, Enforcement actions have been taken domestically.

Types of drugs for which COPPs may be issued

- Approved drug products
- Active pharmaceutical ingredients (API)
- Over the counter drug (OTC) products
- Unapproved drug products
- Homeopathic drugs

Who can Apply for COPP?

- A complete application for export certification must be submitted by the company who exports the drug.
- The certification is intended for a drug which: meets the applicable requirements of the Act or FDA 801(e) (1) requirements.

Process to apply for a COPP

a. Submit Form no. 3613b – located on the FDA internet

www.fda.gov/downloads/AboutFDA/Reports_Manuals_Forms/Forms/UCM052388

b) Requirements for COPP application:

- Applicant Contact information
- Trade name (the product's brand name)
- Bulk substance Generic name
- Name of Applicant
- Status of product license holder
- Listing of manufacturing location on COPP
- Complete Manufacturing Facility Address
- Facility Registration Number
- Importing countries
- Authorization to release information
- Number of certificates requested
- Marketing status in the exporting country

Attachments to COPP

- Two sets of attachments required for one country (one set to attach to the certificate package and one set for FDA files).
- Attachments must not be more than five pages per certificate.
- Applicant is responsible for consulting with the importing country to determine the type of the information required.

Process Time

- Drugs in compliance are normally issued within 20 government working days of receipt of complete and an accurate COPP application

Certificates may not be issued

- Returned- Missing information application with a letter identifying the missing information.
- Rejected- Manufacturing facilities are not in compliance with good manufacturing practices (GMPs).
- Denied- Drug products are not compliance as per regulation (e.g. misbranded drug)

Ribbons on COPPs

- Coloured ribbons designate the type of COPP:

Red: Approved drug product, API, OTC marketed as per monograph, and export only drugs.
Blue: Unapproved drug product not marketed in the country.
Yellow: Drug manufactured with foreign manufacturing sites.
Expiration of COPP

- Certificate expires on 2 years from the notarization date or as noted.
- After expiry date, a new COPP application has to be submitted.

Benefits

- To grow business in foreign country, necessary to obtain the COPP certificates by pharmaceutical companies.

Summary

- Know the requirements of the importing country prior to submitting an application while obtaining COPP.
- Complete Application Form no. 3613b.

Submission of required documentation.

Regulatory requirements and approval procedures for New Drugs

New Drug Application (NDA) is an application submitted preclinical and clinical test data for analysing the drug information and description of manufacturing procedures. After agency received the NDA possibilities:

1. Approval
2. Approvable
3. Not Approvable

Drug Development Teams:

Drug development is the process of bringing a new pharmaceutical drug to the market once a lead compound has been identified through the process of drug discovery. The process of drug discovery and development is very long and needs around 10-12 years which includes the close interaction of large number of scientific disciplines.

Drug Development Team Responsibilities

1. Planning research studies to further characterization of drug candidate.
2. Integration of new research results with previously generated data.
3. Preparation of detailed drug development plan (designing the Development milestones, generating timelines for completion and defining critical path).
4. Reviewing research results from experiments conducted by various scientific disciplines.
5. Monitoring the status of ongoing research studies and modifying the plan as per new data.
6. Comparing research results and development status of drug molecules of competitors.

The new drug approval is of two-phase process:

First phase for clinical trials and second phase for marketing authorization of drug. Firstly, non-clinical studies of a drug are completed to ensure efficacy and safety, and then application for conduct of clinical trials is submitted to the competent authority of the concerned country. Thereafter, the clinical trials can be conducted (phase I to phase IV). These studies are performed to ensure the efficacy, safety and optimizing the dose of drug in human beings.

After the completion of clinical studies of the drug, then an application to the competent authority of the concerned country for the approval of drug for marketing is submitted. The competent authority reviews the application and approve the drug for marketing only if the drug is found to be safe and effective in human being or the drug have more desirable effect as compare to the adverse effect. Even after the approval of new drug, government should monitor its safety due to appearance of some side effects, when it is used in larger population. The interactions with other drugs, which were not assessed in a pre-marketing research trial and its adverse effects.

NON-CLINICAL DRUG DEVELOPMENT

Pre-clinical trial:

A laboratory test for a novel drug or a new medical device is usually done on animal subjects, to see if the hoped-for treatment really works and if it is safe to test on humans. It includes various studies,

- in silico: via computer simulation
- in vivo: within the living
- in vitro: within the glass (outside the living organism)

This process of non-clinical development of medicine is very complex, time consuming and regulatory driven.

The primary aims of the non-clinical development phase is to analyse and determine which candidate has the greatest probability of success, assess its safety, and raise firm scientific foundations before transition to the clinical development phase.

Pharmacology: Study of effects of chemical substances on living systems. It holds all the aspects of drug discovery, ranging from details of interaction between drug molecule and its target to consequences of placing the drug in the market.

Selectivity Testing: It consists of two main stages i.e., screening for selectivity and Binding assay. To determine the potency of drug, the selectivity of a compound for a chosen molecular target needs to be assessed.

Pharmacological Profiling: This includes the determination of pharmacodynamics effect of new compound, either on in-vitro models or in-vivo models.

SAFETY PHARMACOLOGY

This includes the scientific evaluation and study of potentially life-threatening pharmacological effects of a potential drug which is unrelated to the desired therapeutic effect and therefore may present a hazard.

- These tests are conducted at doses not too much in excess of the intended clinical dose.
- Safety pharmacology seeks to identify unanticipated effects of new drugs on major organ function
- It is aimed at detecting possible undesirable or dangerous effects of exposure of the drug in therapeutic doses

TOXICOLOGICALAPPROACHES TO DRUG DISCOVERY

Acute Toxicity: Acute toxicity studies: at least two species, usually mice and rats using the same route as intended for humans. In addition, at least two more routes should be used to ensure systemic absorption of the drug; this route may depend on the nature of the drug. Mortality should be looked for up to 72 hours after parenteral administration and up to 7 days after oral administration. The symptoms, signs and mode of death should be reported, with appropriate macroscopic and microscopic findings where necessary.

Long-Term Toxicity: These studies should be carried out in at least two mammalian species and out of these two mammalian species one should be a non-rodent. The duration of study will depend on the factor that whether the application is for marketing permission or for clinical trial, and in the latter case, on the phases of trials. If a species is known to metabolize the drug in the same way as humans, it should be preferred in long-term toxicity studies. The drug should be administered 7 days a week by the route intended for clinical use in humans.

REGULATORY ORGANIZATIONS IN DIFFERENT COUNTRIES

USFDA (Unites States)

CDSCO- Central drugs standard control organization (India)

EMEA- European Agency for the evaluation of medicinal products (European Union)

MoH (Sri Lanka)

DDA- Department of drug Administration (Nepal)

DIFFERENT TYPES OF DRUG APPLICATIONS THAT CAN BE SUBMITTED TO FDA

- IND (Investigational New Drug Application
- NDA (New Drug Application)
- ANDA (Abbreviated New Drug Application)
- BLA (Biologic License Application)

FDA is responsible for protecting and promoting public health. The IND application should provide high quality preclinical data to justify the testing of the drug in humans. Almost 85% of drugs are subjected to clinical trials, for which IND applications are filed.

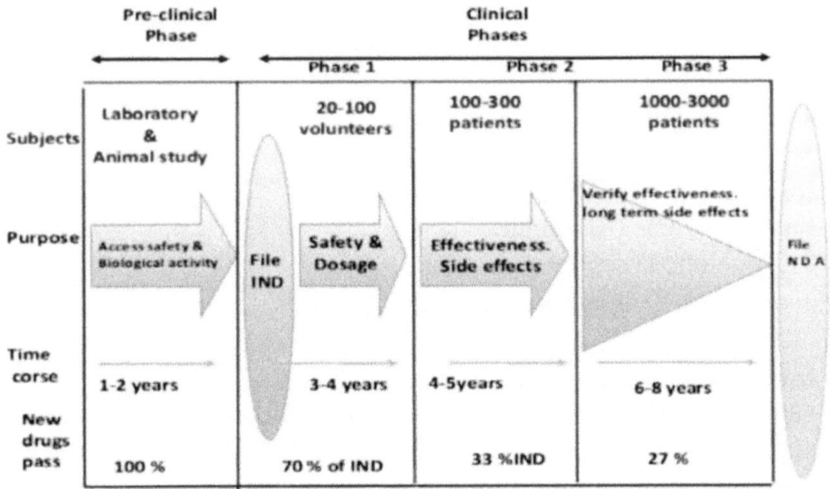

Investigational New Drug Application (INDA)

Its application filed to FDA in order to start clinical trials in humans if the drug was found to be safe form the report of Preclinical trials.

A pre-IND meeting can be arranged with the FDA to discuss a number of issues:

- The design of Animal research.
- Protocol for conducting the Clinical trials.
- Review the chemistry, manufacturing, and control of the investigational drug.

IND application is filled to provide the data showing that it is reasonable to begin tests of a new drug on humans. During a new drug's early preclinical development, the sponsor's primary goal is to determine if the product is reasonably safe for initial use in humans and if the compound exhibits pharmacological activity that justifies commercial development. When a product is identified viable candidate for further development, the sponsor then focuses on collecting the data and information necessary to establish that the product will not expose humans to unreasonable risks when used in limited, early-stage clinical studies.

FDA's role in the development of a new drug begins when the drug's sponsor having screened the new molecule for pharmacological activity and acute toxicity potential in animals, wants to test its diagnostic. At that point, the molecule changes in legal status under the Federal Food, Drug, and Cosmetic Act and becomes a new drug subject to specific requirements of the drug regulatory system.

TYPES OF IND APPLICATIONS

- Investigator IND application
- Emergency Use IND application
- Treatment IND application
- Screening IND application

Investigator IND application:

Submitted by a physician who both initiates and conducts an investigation, and under whose immediate direction the investigational drug is administered or dispensed. Physician might submit a research IND to propose studying an unapproved drug, or an approved product for a new indication or in a new patient population.

Emergency Use IND

- Allows FDA to authorize use of an experimental drug in an emergency situation.

- Does not allow time for submission of an IND in accordance with 21CFR , Sec. 312.23 or Sec. 312.34 .

Treatment IND:

Submitted for experimental drugs showing promise in clinical testing for serious or immediately life-threatening conditions while the final clinical work is conducted and the FDA review takes place.

Laws, regulations, Policies, Procedures

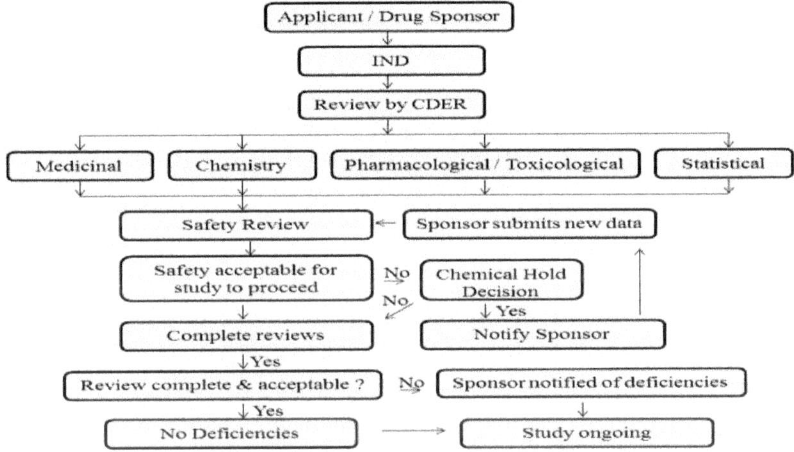

Investigational New Drug Application (IND)

Code Of Federal Regulations (CFR):

The final regulations published in the Federal Register (daily published record of proposed rules, final rules, meeting notices, etc.) are collected in the CFR.

The CFR is divided into 50 titles that represent broad areas subject to Federal regulations. The FDA's portion of the CFR interprets the The Federal Food, Drug, and Cosmetic Act and related statutes. Section 21 of the CFR contains most regulations pertaining to food and drugs.

21CFR Part 312	Investigational New Drug Application
21CFR Part 314	INDA and NDA Applications for FDA Approval to Market a New Drug (New Drug Approval)
21CFR Part 316	Orphan Drugs
21CFR Part 58	Good Lab Practice for Nonclinical Laboratory [Animal] Studies
21CFR Part 50	Protection of Human Subjects
21CFR Part 56	Institutional Review Boards
21CFR Part 201	Drug Labeling
21CFR Part 54	Financial Disclosure by Clinical Investigators

INVESTIGATOR'S BROCHURE (IB) It is a compilation of the clinical and non-clinical data on the investigational product that are relevant to the study of the product in human subject.

- Provide information to the investigators and others involved in the trial such as the dose, dose frequency/interval, methods of administration and safety monitoring procedures.
- Provides insight to support the clinical management of the study subjects during the course of the clinical trial. The information should be presented in a concise and simple manner.

Contents of Investigator's Brochure:

1. Table of contents.
2. Summary not exceeding 2 pages, highlighting
3. Introduction: Chemical name, API, pharmacological class, anticipated therapeutic/diagnostic indication(s). General approach to be followed in evaluating the IP.
4. Description of I.P.: Physical, chemical and pharmaceutical properties of I.P. Storage and handling of I.P. and clinical data of IP.
5. Non-clinical studies: The results of all relevant non-clinical pharmacology, toxicology, pharmacokinetic, and investigational product metabolism studies should be provided in summary form. The information provided may include: Species tested, Number of sexes in each group, Unit dose, Dose interval, Route of administration and Duration of dosing.

6. Effects in Humans: A thorough discussion of the known effects of the investigational product(s) in humans should be provided, including information on pharmacokinetics, metabolism, Pharmacodynamics, dose response, safety, efficacy, and other pharmacological activities. (a) Pharmacokinetics and Product Metabolism in Humans.

7. Summary of Data and Guidance for the Investigator: This section should contain non-clinical.

NEW DRUG APPLICATION (NDA)

If clinical studies confirm that a new drug is relatively safe and effective and will not pose unreasonable risk to patients, the manufacturer files a New Drug Application, the actual request to manufacture and sell the drug in the United States.

Aim of NDA:

- Safety and effectiveness of drug,
- Benefits overweigh risks,
- Is the drug's proposed labelling appropriate, and what should it contain?
- Are the methods used in manufacturing (GMP) the drug and the controls used to maintain the drug's quality adequate to preserve the drug's identity, strength, quality, and purity?

- Once the application is submitted, the FDA has 60 days to conduct a preliminary review which will assess whether the NDA is "sufficiently complete to permit a substantive review". If everything is found to be acceptable, the FDA will decide if the NDA will get a standard or accelerated review and communicate the acceptance of the application and their review choice in another communication known as the 74- day letter.

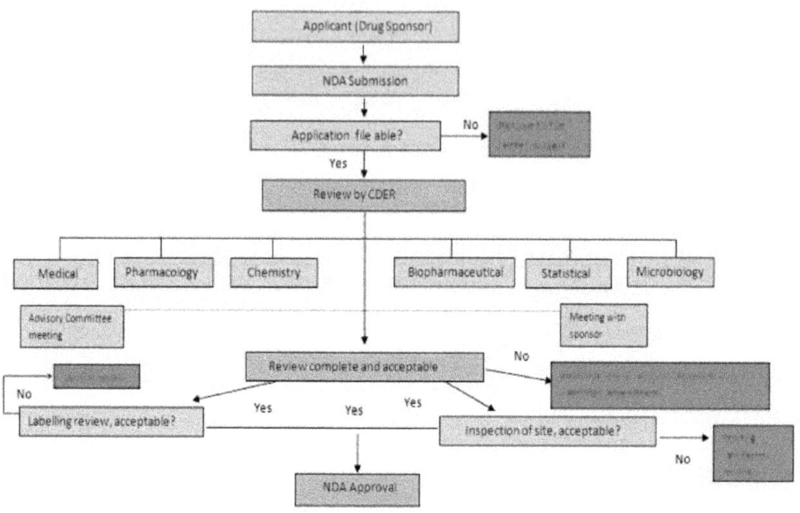

BIO EQUIVALENCE STUDIES

BE studies are essential to ensure uniformity in standards of quality, efficacy and safety of pharmaceutical products so that reasonable assurance can be provide for the various products containing same active ingredient, marketed by different licensees are clinically equivalent and interchangeable. Both Bioavailability and Bioequivalence focus on release of drug substance from its dosage form and subsequent absorption in circulation. Similar approaches to measure bioavailability should be followed in demonstrating bioequivalence.

Bioavailability: Rate and extent to which the active ingredient or active moiety is absorbed from a drug product and becomes available at the site of action.

Equivalence: It is a relative term that compares drug products with respect to a specific characteristic or function or to a defined set of standards.

Abbreviated New Drug Application (ANDA)

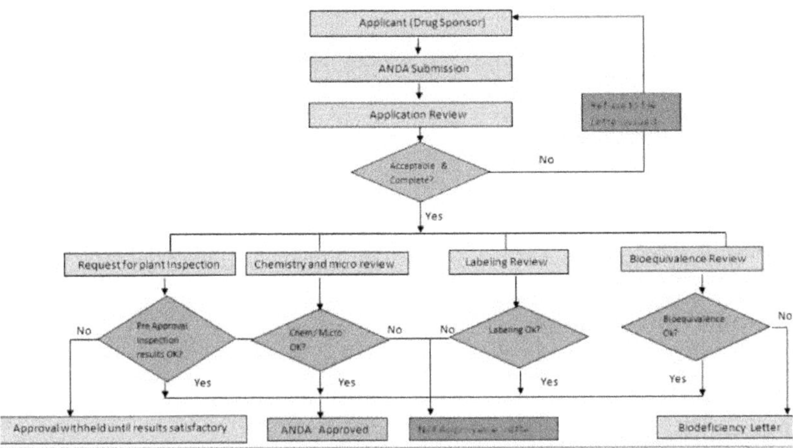

It's an application made for approval of Generic Drugs. The sponsor is not required to reproduce the clinical studies that were done for the original, brand name product. Instead, generic drug manufacturers must demonstrate that their product is the same as, and bioequivalent to, a previously approved brand name product.

CLINICAL RESEARCH PROTOCOLS

It is a complete written description of and scientific rationale for a research activity involving human subjects. Sufficient information is to be gathered on the quality of the non- clinical safety to conduct the protocol and health authority/ethics committee approval is granted in the country where approval of the drug or device is sought.

The clinical trial design and objectives are written into a document called a clinical trial protocol. It is a document that states the background, objectives, rationale, design, methodology and statistical considerations of the study. It also states the conditions under which the study shall be performed and managed. Look for better ways to prevent disease in people who never had the disease or to prevent a disease from returning.

CLINICAL RESEARCH PROTOCOLS

- To clarify the research question.
- To compile existing knowledge.
- To formulate a hypothesis and objectives.
- To decide about a study design.

- To clarify ethical considerations.
- To apply for funding.
- To have a guideline and tool for the research team.

Parts of the Protocol:

1. Title Page.
2. Signature Page.
3. Content Page.
4. List of Abbreviations.
5. Introduction/Abstract.
6. Objectives.
7. Background/Rationale.
8. Eligibility Criteria.
9. Study Design/Methods
10. Safety/Adverse Events.
11. Regulatory Guidance.
12. Statistical Section
13. Human Subjects Protection/Informed Consent.

DATA PRESENTATION FOR FDA SUBMISSIONS

Study data standards describe a standard way to exchange clinical and non-clinical Study data. These standards provide a consistent general framework for organizing study data, including templates for datasets, standard names for variables; identify appropriate controlled terminology and standard ways of doing calculations with common variables. Data standards also help FDA receive, process, review, and archive submissions more efficiently and effectively.

FDA has been working towards a standardized approach to capture, receive and analyze study data. Standardization of study data is vital to integrate pre-marketing study data and post-marketing safety data to improve public health and patient safety. Central to this vision is the creation of an enterprise data infrastructure (Janus) within FDA to improve the management of all structured scientific data.

MANAGEMENT OF CLINICAL STUDIES

Clinical trial management is most simply defined as the process that an organization follows to ensure that quality (defined as minimized risks and clean data) is delivered efficiently and punctually. It refers to a standards-driven process that a project manager initiates and follows in order to successfully manage clinical trial sites, clinical research associates, and workflow by using clinical trial management tools or software prolonged timelines and heavy costs related to large trials have been prompted a new focus on more efficient clinical trial management.

It is possible to dramatically reduce the total cost of a clinical trial by 60% - 90% without compromising the scientific validity of the results.

Life Cycle of Clinical Trial Project:

A more accurate control, regardless of the therapeutic area or trial stages is ensured by typically breaking down the life cycle of each clinical trial project into 4 phases:

- Conceptual,
- Planning,
- Implementation,
- Analysis.

Clinical Trial Protocol: A protocol is a document that describes the purpose, design, methodology, statistical considerations and organization of a study, and provides basic information and rationale for the clinical study. The contents that should be present in the protocol are described by the GCP. The protocol writing is a task for one person, usually the principal investigator, not a committee.

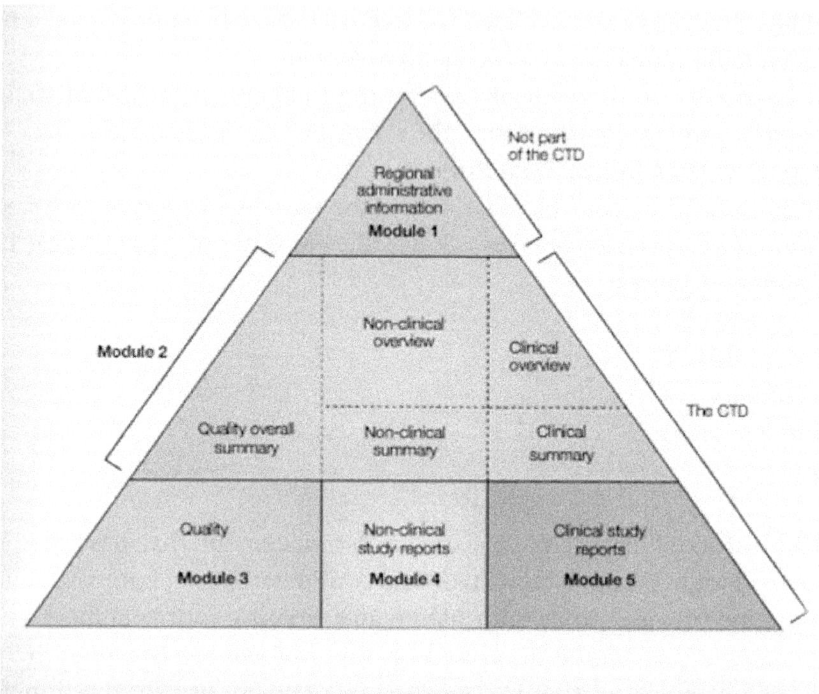

- There are various challenges of Project management in clinical trials. Clinical trials all need the same coordinated processes and systems, irrespective of the size, scope, costs, or period. The key challenge is then to implement and maintain effective management systems and techniques in response to the needs of the trial project.

- Manufacturing, importing, or conducting a clinical trial requires permission from the licensing authority through a Form 44 application. The application follows international submission requirements of a Common Technical Document (CTD) and has five modules.

Conclusion: The Drug approvals in the US, Europe & India are the most demanding in the world. The primary purpose of the rules governing medicinal products in US, Europe & India is to safeguard public health. It is the role of public regulatory authorities to ensure that pharmaceutical companies comply with regulations. There are legislations that require drugs to be developed, tested, trailed, and manufactured in accordance to the guidelines so that they are safe and patient's well - being is protected.

www.ingramcontent.com/pod-product-compliance
Ingram Content Group UK Ltd.
Pitfield, Milton Keynes, MK11 3LW, UK
UKHW022021190726
13853UKWH00005B/2041

9 798889 353706